EVERYDAY
CHI KUNG

WITH MASTER LAM

'This is the gateway to indescribable marvels'
– Lao Tse, the Tao Teh Ching

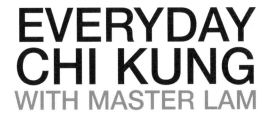

EVERYDAY
CHI KUNG
WITH MASTER LAM

15-minute routines to build energy,
boost immunity and banish stress

Master Lam Kam-Chuen

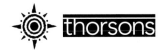

Thorsons
An Imprint of HarperCollins*Publishers*
77–85 Fulham Palace Road,
Hammersmith, London W6 8JB

The website address is:
www.thorsonselement.com

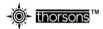 thorsons™

and *Thorsons* are trademarks of
HarperCollins*Publishers* Ltd

First published by Thorsons 2004

10 9 8 7 6 5 4 3 2 1

© Master Lam Kam-Chuen 2004

Master Lam Kam-Chuen asserts the moral right to
be identified as the author of this work

A catalogue record of this book
is available from the British Library

ISBN 0 00 716102 6

Photographs © Guy Hearn

Printed and bound in Great Britain by
Martins the Printers Limited, Berwick upon Tweed

Contents

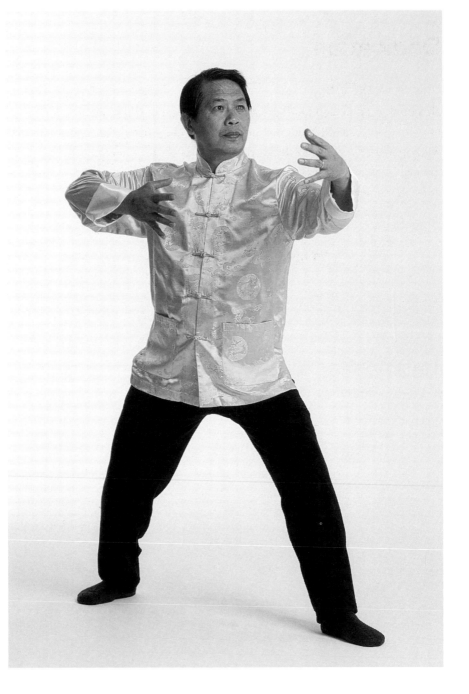

Dedication

This book is dedicated to all the masters of the art of Chi Kung. In particular it is dedicated to Grand Master Wang Xiang Zhai, who opened this art up to the world in the last century, and to my own master, Professor Yu Yong Nian in Beijing, who first introduced me to the art of Zhan Zhuang Chi Kung.

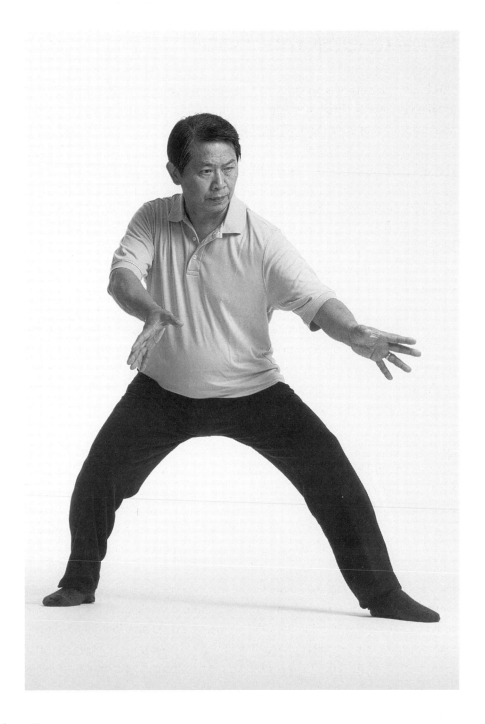

How to Use this Book

This book is a step-by-step guide to Chi Kung practice. It is carefully designed to take you slowly through the foundations of this art, giving you the instructions you need at each stage along the way.

The structure of this book follows the way Chi Kung students have been taught by their masters over the centuries. Each student had to develop a solid foundation, appropriate for them and for their health, before moving on to the next level of training. That kind of highly individual attention is not possible in a book. But the instructions in these pages have been structured by Master Lam so that, if you follow them carefully, you will progress safely on the path of Chi Kung study.

For this reason, you will find it helpful to work with this book by starting at the beginning and moving methodically through to the end. A classical master would never introduce a beginner to advanced practices, because the student might suffer internal harm from a sudden burst of energy. Centuries of experience have shown that you need to begin at the beginning.

You might feel like dipping in and out of the book, trying out the various exercises at random. However, a better approach would be to treat this book as your teacher. You can follow it as if Master Lam was giving you an ordinary class. In fact, you could just imagine that he was coming to your home, like a personal trainer, to lead you through 15 minutes of guided Chi Kung practice. The way to do this is to work through the book, step by step, from beginning to end.

It's a good idea to practise a little Chi Kung often, ideally every day, but don't worry if you can only manage two or three times a week, or at first only once or twice. You will still enjoy the full benefits of Chi Kung when you are practising and it will just take you a little longer to progress through the programme. Try, at any rate, to develop a routine so that you get into the habit of practising regularly.

The book is divided into different sections, each building on the one before. It begins with a short outline of the history and benefits of Chi Kung (*pages 4–10*). A little history is helpful because it is important that you understand how these practices have evolved. What you are doing now, in the 21st century, is the result of at least 27 previous centuries of investigation, study and practice, almost entirely handed down from person to person over the generations.

At the end of the opening section there is important advice on what to do before you begin your daily practice (*see pages 10–11*). Please read that carefully.

The first stage of your training will be in the preliminary practices known as Gathering your Chi. These are presented on pages 14–33. It's always important to do these warm-ups, just the way we do warm-ups before any kind of exercise. And it's just as important to do the short concluding practices at the end of your training.

The next stage of your training is Building your Chi. This is presented on pages 36–83. It is sometimes surprising to beginners to find that these high-energy exercises involve no movement. The reason they work is explained in the introduction, where you'll find out about the history of this art and the way energy works in the human body.

The following sections train you in Guiding Your Chi (*see pages 86–101*) and Increasing Your Chi (*see pages 104–55*).

Throughout the book there are structured schedules for your training. These take you through six levels, which guide your daily practice for your first year. At the end (*see pages 159–63*) there are sample schedules that will enable you to structure your own training after that. They can also be adapted for daily life, whether at work, home or if you happen to be ill and in bed (*see pages 156–8*).

Almost all the practices in this book can be done sitting or standing. However, this flexibility applies only to advanced Chi Kung practitioners. When starting your first year of Chi Kung practice, you are strongly advised to follow the sequence of sitting and standing positions presented by your teacher, which in this case is this book. Thus, Levels One through Four are all practised while sitting. The standing practices are introduced gradually, once a week, in Levels Five and Six.

If you decide to go further in your Chi Kung practice, try to find a qualified Chi Kung instructor from whom you can receive personal instruction. If you have a serious medical condition you are advised to consult your doctor before undertaking Chi Kung practice. Nevertheless, you can be confident that the advice in this book is set out so that if you follow the instructions and are careful not to overdo anything, you will be in safe hands.

The book concludes (*see pages 166–87*) with advice and practices on relaxation and a short set of exercises you can do when travelling. The advice on relaxation is extremely important. It is so important that you would normally expect to find it at the beginning of a book like this. So, if you really can't resist jumping ahead, the first thing you'll find at the back of the book is Master Lam telling you to relax – sound advice for all levels!

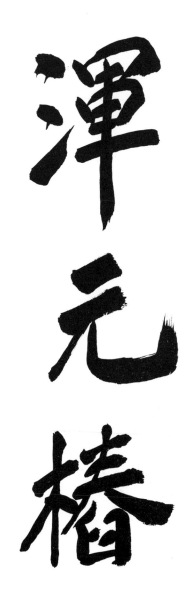

CHAPTER ONE

THE ART OF
CHI KUNG

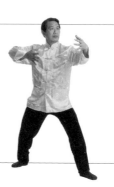

In an era of increasing speed and anxiety, more and more people are turning to the quiet power of Chi Kung. This ancient art is more now widely practised than at any previous time in history, as people seek an antidote to the stress and disorder of contemporary life.

Chi Kung (pronounced 'chee gung') literally means energy exercise. 'Chi' is the Chinese term for energy. 'Kung' means exercise. When we think of exercise, we often think of activities that use up energy. This type of exercise is different. It increases and transforms energy. The classical character for chi has two elements. On top are five strokes that appear to resemble a cooking pot with a handle. Underneath are four strokes that flick upward like little flames. The whole image represents the process of cooking over a fire. The calligraphy is an excellent symbol for the transformation of energy. You'll find it on top of each right hand page of this book.

The Chi Kung system you'll be learning is one of the most powerful forms of exercise ever invented. Yet it involves almost no movement. You will be introduced to a series of postures that have been carefully developed over the centuries.

This remarkable system is known in Chinese as Zhan Zhuang (pronounced 'jam jong'). It means 'to stand like a tree'. Like a tree, you are completely still, rooted to the power of the earth and completely open to the energy of the universe.

You can think of Chi Kung as a mighty tree itself. Its history stretches over the centuries of Chinese civilization. It is a tree with many branches. One branch is connected with the tradition of the Tao – 'the Way' – the ancient spiritual tradition of living in harmony with nature. Another branch is associated with the Buddhist tradition that was introduced to China from India. For both the Taoist and Buddhist traditions, Chi Kung offered a powerful method of clearing the mind and strengthening the nervous system.

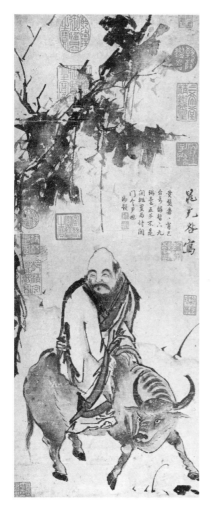

Lao Tse

Chi Kung's cleansing and toning effect on the vital organs was naturally of interest to China's earliest medical specialists and was integrated into the developing tradition that stressed the many ways in which people can take responsibility for their own health. And because it so dramatically increased the inner power of those who practised it, Chi Kung became an indispensable component of the martial arts tradition.

These days, however, to practise Chi Kung you don't need to be a philosopher, doctor or martial artist. You don't need to be a Taoist or a Buddhist. You don't need to be Chinese or take up the study of ancient history. Chi Kung has become a part of world culture. It is practised by millions of people who are simply seeking a safe and well-tested method of personal health care.

The Chi Kung lineage

The art of cultivating internal energy has been passed down in an unbroken line of masters and students that goes back 27 centuries. In one of the earliest-known texts of Chinese civilization, *The Natural Way of Life*, the philosopher Guan Tse described energy as the foundation of all human activity. The great sage, Lao Tse, who is said to have composed the world-famous collection of verses, the *Tao Teh Ching*, described early Chi Kung practice in these words: 'Standing alone and unchanging is the source of all power. The energy of the cosmos is inexhaustible'. The deep influence of Chi Kung is reflected in one of the world's earliest medical manuals, *The Yellow Emperor's Classic of Internal Medicine*, which speaks of the remarkable health and longevity of the sages who preserved their 'vital spirit'.

Records from the first century of our common era show that the standing practices of Chi Kung were embraced by both the Taoist and Buddhist traditions in China. The aim was to develop high levels of internal energy that could be projected outward when needed – a practice that could be used for healing and the contemplative arts.

Over the succeeding centuries these practices were preserved as family secrets, normally passed from father to son. It was not until the 20th century that they were taught publicly. The person credited with making the art of Chi Kung accessible to the public was Grand Master Wang Xiang Zhai (pronounced 'Wang Shang Jai'). Initially introduced to the art by his uncle, Master Guo Yun Sin, the young Wang Xiang Zhai travelled throughout China meeting and studying under the great practitioners of his time. Eventually, by the mid-1920s he began teaching, first in Shanghai and later in Beijing. For the benefit of his many students, Grand Master Wang composed poems to guide them on the path of Chi Kung practice – attempting to convey in words the inner experience of this art:

> To master the quintessence of this art, begin with standing still.
> As if it were from high in the clouds, Your breathing should be deep,
> smooth and gentle. You are going through a furnace:
> Everything mental and physical is tempered and moulded –
> Preserving the heavenly wisdom and maintaining the state of quiescence,
> You are ready to act in response to all possible situations.

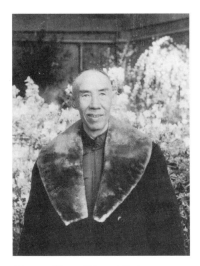

Master Wang Xiang Zhai

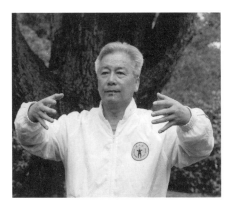

Professor Yu Yong Nian

One of Grand Master Wang's first students was a dental surgeon, Professor Yu Yong Nian. The health benefits of Chi Kung were so impressive that he introduced it at the hospital where he worked. This lead to a major medical conference in 1956 that introduced methods of Chi Kung treatment to medical facilities throughout China. As one of the world's leading authorities on Chi Kung, his influence extended not only throughout China, but internationally. I first learned of Professor Yun from a newspaper article in the 1960s, when I was still studying classical Chinese arts in Hong Kong. For years it was only possible for me to correspond with Professor Yu until, towards the end of China's Cultural Revolution, I was finally able to travel to Beijing and be accepted as a one of his students. Even though I now live and teach in the West, I continue to respect the classical tradition of the master–student relationship, returning regularly to China to practise with, and learn from, Professor Yu's lifetime of experience in this art.

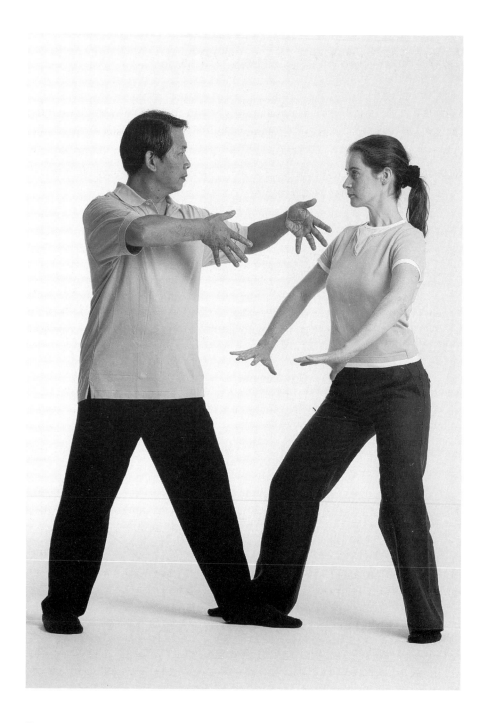

Understanding Chi Kung

Why is a system that involves almost no external movement a powerful form of exercise? Why do sitting and standing still in the various positions make you feel refreshed and energized? If Chi Kung generates high levels of energy, why does it calm the nervous system? These are questions I am most often asked about the Zhan Zhuang system of Chi Kung.

The basis of understanding Chi Kung is an appreciation of energy. From the earliest natural scientists of Chinese civilization down to the quantum physicists of our own era, there has been a tradition of understanding all phenomena as an expression of energy. In Chinese, this energy, or life force, is known as 'chi'. It is not only the basis of human life but is none other than the vast force field that gives birth to, and sustains, everything in the universe – visible and invisible.

The unobstructed flow of this energy is what enables life to flourish. If the flow of energy is blocked, then, like stagnant water, energy putrifies. What blocks the flow of chi within our bodies is tension – the subtle effect of mental strain and its imprint on our muscles and nerves. Chi Kung practice relieves this tension and clears the blockages.

The distinct feature of the Zhan Zuang system of still postures presented in this book is that you increase the circulation of blood in the body (as with conventional external exercises) without becoming breathless. In fact, your breathing tends to become deeper, guaranteeing a higher volume of oxygen in circulation throughout your entire system.

This heightened flow of energy automatically strengthens and calms your nervous system because this inner relaxation and power is your natural state. What we mistake for a normal life is in fact the anxiety and discomfort we experience as a result of living with diminished and obstructed energy.

Is Chi Kung a form of meditation? Many people ask me this question. The answer is 'yes' and 'no'. Zhan Zhuang is often described as standing meditation. It calms and clears your mind. On the other hand, many people associate meditation with mind control. This is definitely not what you are taught to do when practising this style of Chi Kung, and please do not try mixing in other disciplines when you are doing your daily training (for example, don't be tempted to add a religious visualization). Just allow the energy of your mind to roam at will. Please keep your eyes open and don't try to shut out the sounds of life around you. You are learning to stand like a tree – a powerhouse of energy, at home on the earth surrounded by the energy of the universe.

Some people may wonder why, in the Sealing position (see pages 30–3), you place your right hand, palm up, on top of your left hand, also palm up. *(Note: when you stand in the sealing position you bring your hands flat against the belly so the left palm folds over the back of the right hand.)* In various Chi Kung systems, the hand position may be different for women and men, but here you are advised to place your right palm uppermost, regardless of your gender. The reason is that in this system your self-healing powers are being trained. Your right hand will be the instrument for your healing and therefore rests on top, holding an imaginary crystal sphere, close to the internal energy reservoir in your lower abdomen. By adopting this position, you are secretly developing the powerful connection between that hand and your chi reservoir.

Before you Begin

Normally Chi Kung is practised in the morning. If you do it before breakfast, then it's a good idea to drink a little warm water (not tea or coffee) before you start. You can have your breakfast any time after your morning practice. If you have breakfast first, then allow a short gap before you start your training. If you do your training at night, it is best to do it in a room with a light on. Preferably there should be a source of fresh air in the room. If it is not possible to open a window, avoid a room where the air is stale.

You can try practising Chi Kung before going to bed. Some people may find that they sleep extremely well as a result. Others may find that they feel too energized to sleep – in which case, it is better to train in the mornings only.

You can practise Chi Kung outdoors – the way it has been practised in China for centuries. But don't practise outdoors when it is windy or raining.

If you are feeling sad, extremely frustrated or angry you should calm yourself by going for a walk or talking to a close friend – it is best not to practise Chi Kung when you are under the influence of those troubling emotions. Regular Chi Kung practice, however, will give your greater inner resources to help you in times of distress.

Different people have different sensations when they start to practise Chi Kung. It's common to feel warm, even hot. You might find yourself shaking a little here and then, sometimes a lot as your energy wakes up. And sometimes it hurts to hold the positions, in which case you need to look carefully at the section on relaxation (see pages 167–73). Sometimes it's hard to sit still or stand still, especially if you are always on the go. But please try not to move, even if your nose itches or you feel impatient. Whatever you experience is the result of the deep power of Chi Kung.

If at any time in your Chi Kung practice you feel heat or pressure rushing to your head, start to have a headache, feel dizzy or faint, immediately do the Circling Down movement (see pages 80–1) slowly and carefully six times. Each time, imagine you are standing in a swimming pool, up to your chest in water. You place your arms around a huge inflated ball and slowly press it down into the water, until you are holding it down below your navel. Finish with a chi massage to the face and neck (see pages 78–9). Then completely relax and rest, breathing naturally.

'Internally, we cultivate our natural energy.'

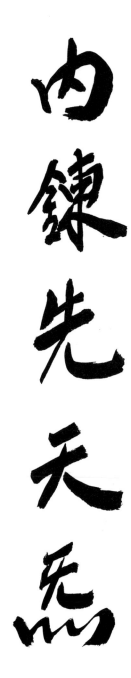

CHAPTER TWO

GATHERING
YOUR CHI

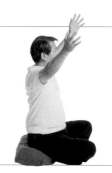

Sitting

Here is something that people often find a little surprising. You can begin Chi Kung by sitting down! This is an extremely powerful way to enter the world of this art because it is so naturally relaxing.

There are four basic sitting positions. You can choose whichever one you prefer and you can also experiment with each one to see which is best suited to your needs. All are equally fine.

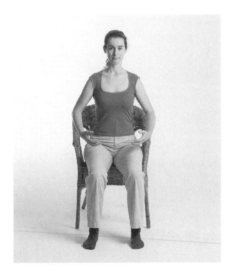

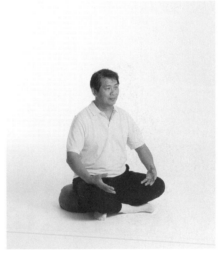

You can sit on a chair. Be sure that your spine is slightly away from the back of the chair, so that you are sitting naturally upright. If you need to use the back of the chair for support, then use it to help you sit upright. Rest your feet flat on the floor.

You can sit on a little stool or firm cushion. Loosely cross your legs in front of you, left leg over right. Try to keep your back upright.

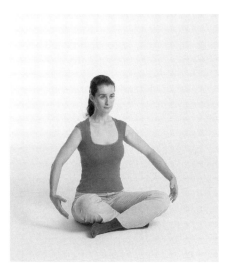

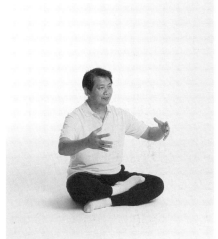

You can sit on the floor, preferably on a rug or carpet for comfort. Loosely cross your legs in front, with your left knee resting on top of your right foot. Try to keep your back upright.

Whether you are sitting on a low stool, support cushion or on the floor, you can cross your legs in the traditional half-lotus position. Your right ankle rests on top of your left thigh. But only practise in this way if you are already accustomed to sitting in this position.

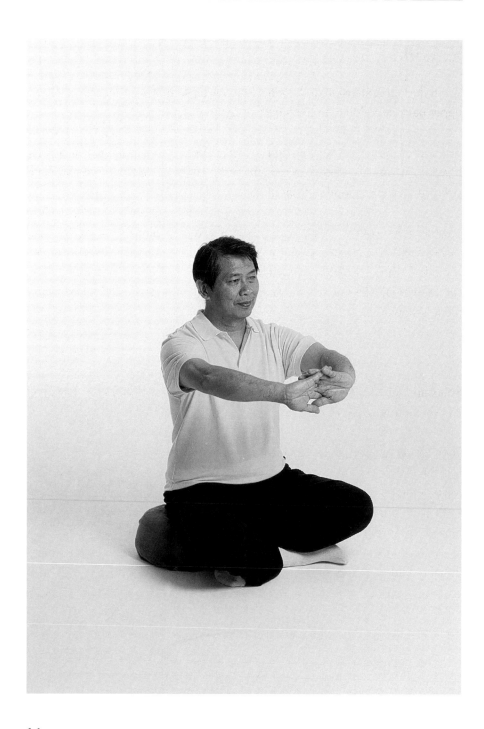

Extending forward

You'll find this extension of the arms releases tension in your shoulders, chest, upper back and along the full length of both arms.

Extend both arms outward in front of your chest. You can clasp your hands together, as shown, or you can have them slightly separated, as if pressing your palms flat against a wall in front of you.

As you extend your arms forward, feel that you are opening your joints in order to lengthen your arms. You feel a little release in your shoulder-blades and shoulders. Then you feel a slight opening of your elbows and wrists. These are subtle internal adjustments: be careful not to strain yourself. The inner movement is slow and gentle.

As you make this inner extension, breathe out.

Relax and let your hands and arms withdraw slightly back toward your chest. As you do this, breathe in.

Then gently and slowly extend forward again, breathing out.

Make a total of eight forward extensions.

Slowly lower both arms when you have completed the eight extensions.

Breathe naturally.

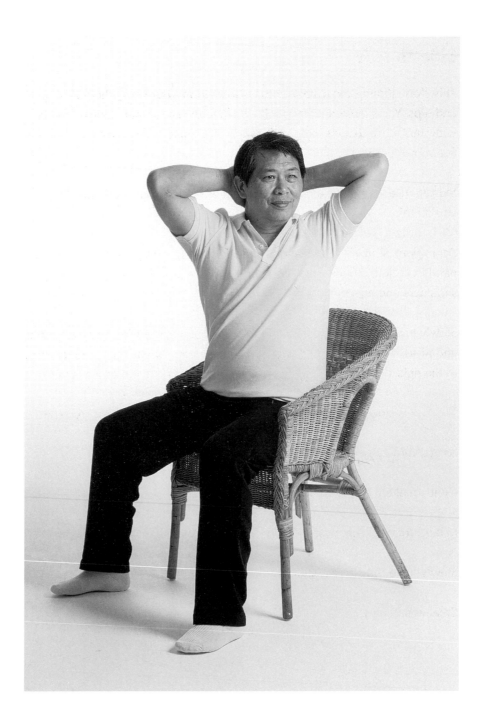

Side to side

This slow, turning movement releases tension in your neck, shoulders, spine and hips. You should do it gradually. Be careful not to strain your back. Begin with small turns to either side and increase the angle of the turn only when you feel more supple.

Slowly raise your arms and grasp your hands behind your head. Breathe in as you do this.

Relax your shoulders and allow them to drop slightly while keeping your hands cradled on the back of your head. Breathe out as you relax your shoulders and turn to the side.

Slowly turn from the hips without changing the alignment of your torso, arms and head. Your entire upper body turns as one unit. If you are a woman, turn to the right diagonal first. If you are a man, turn to the left diagonal first.

The turn is slow and easy-going. Do not turn past the point of any resistance.

As you turn back to face forward, breathe in.

Gently make the same turn to the other diagonal.

Make a total of eight turns, alternating from side to side.

Slowly lower both arms when you have finished.

Breathe naturally.

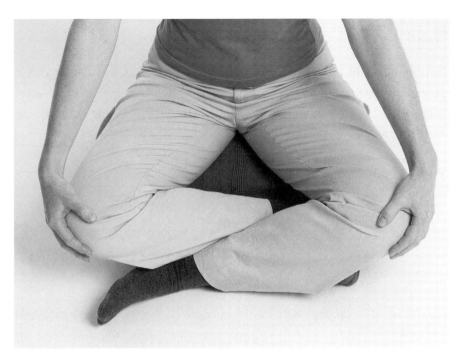

Hands on Knees

Double rubbing

This simple warm-up increases the flow of chi through your knees. Since we want to ensure that chi flows throughout your body, it's all the more important to open the channels around your knees when doing Chi Kung sitting down, especially if you are crossing your legs.

Simply rest both hands on your knees, so that your palms and fingers are comfortably in contact with the area around the joints.

Then gently rub your hands in smooth circles around the whole area of your knees. Your hands circle in an outward direction. Make the massage generous, extending completely around, above and below the knees.

Breathe naturally as your hands circle around the knees twelve times. If you have knee problems, do this massage as many times as you wish.

When you have finished, relax for a moment, with your hands loosely resting on your knees.

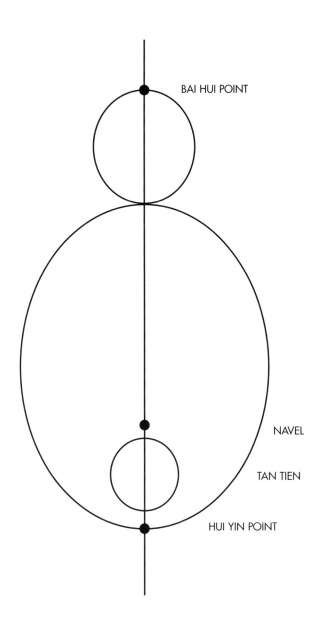

BAI HUI POINT

NAVEL

TAN TIEN

HUI YIN POINT

Energy within you

Before moving on to the next stage, Gathering your Chi (see pages 26–9), it is important to understand the patterns of energy you will be working with in and around your body. This simplified diagram of the torso and head shows five key aspects of the energetic structure of the human body used in Chinese medicine.

The body is organized around a central column, or channel. This runs from the top of the head to the bottom of the torso. Blockages anywhere along this channel seriously disrupt the flow of energy throughout your system. Sitting and standing with your back naturally upright helps prevent or clear such blockages.

At the top of the central channel is the uppermost point of the torso. In Chinese medicine this point is known as Bai Hui, 'the Hundred Meetings'. It is sometimes called the thousand-petalled lotus. This is a particularly sensitive point through which each person's energy field connects with the energy that surrounds them.

At the other end of the channel is the lowermost point of the torso. This is known as the Hui Yin point, 'the Meeting of Yin'. When a person is seated, in particular, this is a powerful point of connection with the supportive energy of the earth.

In the lower abdomen, just below the navel and a short distance into the body, is the energy reservoir known as the Tan Tien. This is pronounced 'dan dyen'. It is sometimes called the 'Field of Elixir', but its more literal translation is 'Sea of Chi'. It is the principal area of energy storage within the entire energetic system of the body.

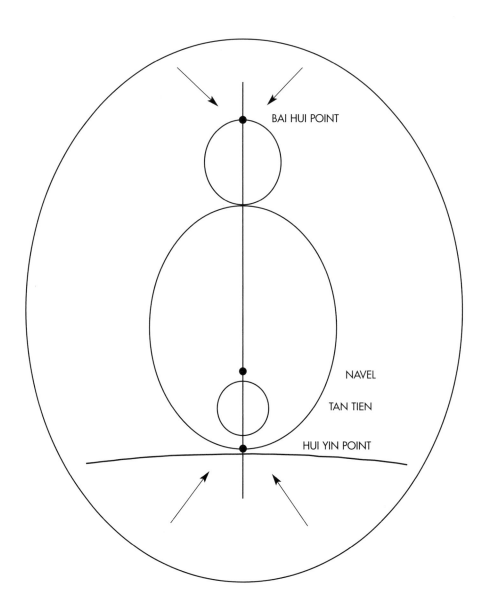

BAI HUI POINT

NAVEL

TAN TIEN

HUI YIN POINT

Energy around you

This simplified model shows how each of us is always at the hub of the energetic forces that surround us at all times. Imagine youself in the middle. You can see your central channel running from the Bai Hui point on the top of the head down to the Hui Yin point at the base of your torso. In the lower abdomen is your Tan Tien.

The outer circle represents the vast and limitless field of energy we call the universe. The line of the circle does not indicate something that is closed or limited. Traditionally a circle is used in Chinese calligraphy to show open space. It is a symbol of limitless possibilities and all possible configurations of energy, visible and invisible.

The long curve below you represents the earth, the vast storehouse of energy that supports all life forms on our planet and is our travelling home in space.

Each human being is an energy field. Because energy attracts energy, we act as magnets for the energy that surrounds us. The arrows represent the constant streams of energy that come to us. The energy from the cosmos, represented by the upper arrows, tends to be more variable and unstable – it is associated with creativity. The energy from the earth, represented by the lower arrows, tends to be more constant and stable – it is associated with power. Your Chi Kung practice enables you to harmonize these two forces within your being.

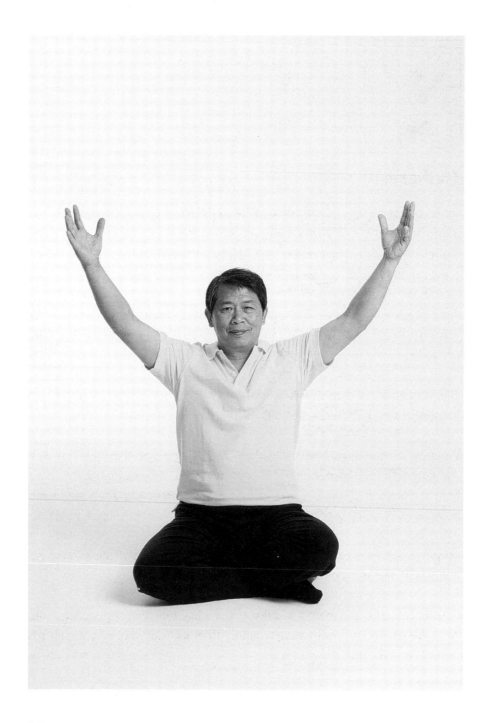

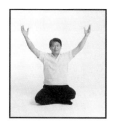 

Gathering

As you sit, in whichever of the seated positions most comfortable for you, direct your attention to your sitting bones. Feel the contact between your body and the floor, stool, support cushion or chair. This is your connection to the energy of the earth.

Then direct your attention to the top of your head, to the central point on the very top of your skull, in line with the tips of your ears. This point is your connection to the energy of the heavens.

Then sit naturally upright for a moment, feeling the rest of your body aligned between these two points. Breathe naturally.

When you sense you are correctly aligned, slowly raise your arms and extend them outward toward the upper diagonals just in front of your body. The arms remain relaxed as you move them into position. Do not force this position into a stretch.

Keeping your arms gently in place, relax your shoulders and chest. The position should feel effortless.

Breathe naturally. The more relaxed you are, while remaining upright and still, the more energy you will naturally gather from the earth below you and the universe around you.

Try remaining in this position for between 30 seconds and one minute.

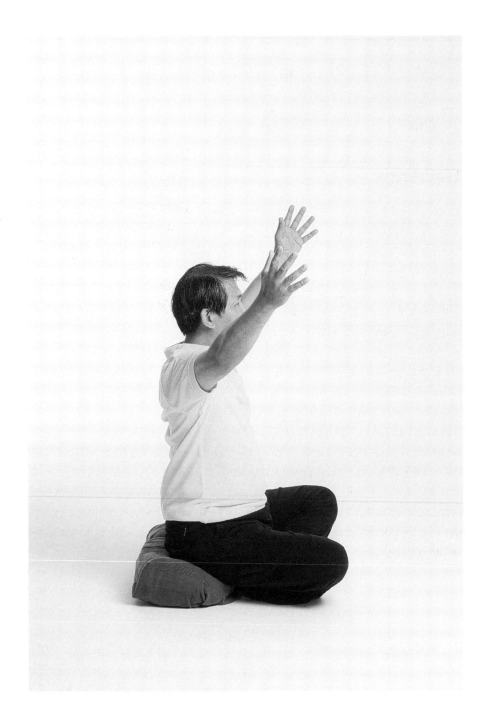

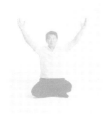 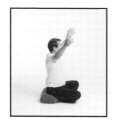

Gathering

While sitting and gathering energy, it is important that your arms be extended slightly forward from your body. If your arms are pulled back in line with your head and shoulders, they will place a strain on your chest and back. This will block the flow of energy.

Although the elbows and wrists appear straight, they are not extended. You should feel they are relaxed, but not limp.

Look straight forward. You feel as if your head is suspended from the central point on the top of your head. You can find the correct point by tracing an arc along your skull with the index finger of each hand up from the tips of both ears until they meet at the top. Feel that this is the uppermost part of the entire structure of your body and relax downward from that point. That will naturally correct the alignment of your head, neck and chin.

Imagine you are holding a large funnel in your arms. It is made of delicate crystal. Into this pours milky white light, known in the Taoist tradition as 'the light of the planets'.

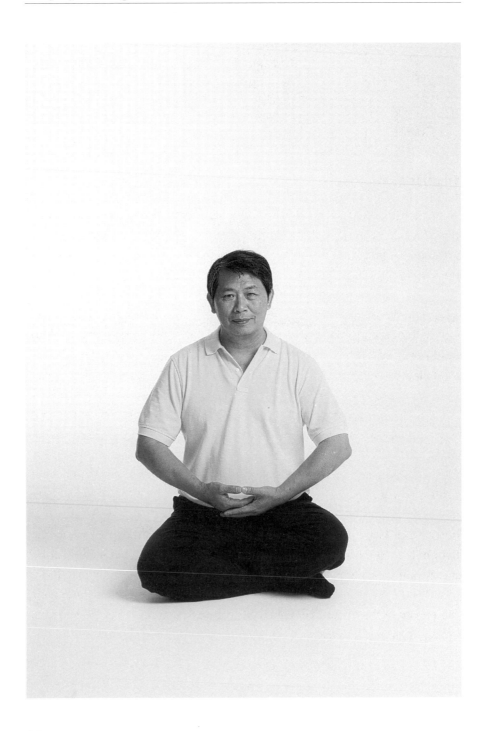

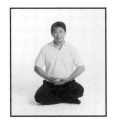 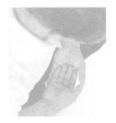

Sealing

After you have spent up to a minute gathering energy, slowly move your hands toward each other and start to lower them down toward your abdomen. Imagine your hands are on top of a large inflated ball that you are gently bringing down to your lap. Breathe slowly out as you do this.

When your hands reach the level of your belly, bring them together in your lap. Turn both palms upward and rest your right hand on top of your left. Find the hand position that is comfortable for you in your lap. You may find it most comfortable to rest your hands on your belly. Do not strain yourself in any way

The tips of your thumbs touch each other lightly – closing the connection between your two hands.

Your shoulders and arms are relaxed as your hands remain comfortably in position in your lap.

This posture has the effect of sealing your accumulated energy into your Tan Tien, in the region of your lower abdomen. You can imagine that the field of energy originally attracted by your outstretched arms has been condensed into a smaller sphere of crystal that you hold in your lap, resting against your belly. The energy of the crystal will naturally be absorbed by the sensitive energetic reservoir below your navel.

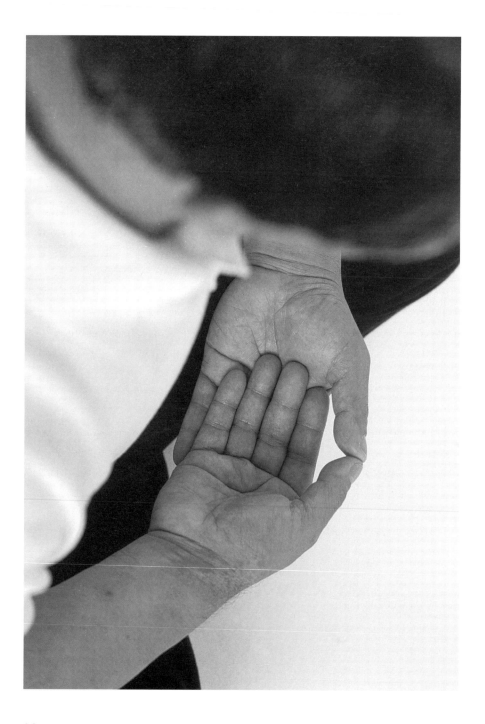

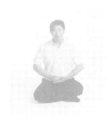 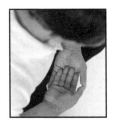

Sealing

As you seal the energy into the reservoir within your abdomen, the back of your right hand rests comfortably on top of the open palm of your left hand.

You may wonder why you place your hands this way. The reason is that you are developing the connection between your right hand and your energy reservoir, for use in Chi Kung healing. Experience shows that the connection is not as strong if your left hand is uppermost, regardless of whether you are left- or right-handed and regardless of whether you are a woman or a man.

Breathe naturally, allowing yourself to settle into this alert, restful position.

Mental relaxation is part of this system. You are not required to think about anything in particular, nor is it a problem if you experience thoughts, feelings or other sensations from time to time. Just allow them to come and go. This is just the spontaneous activity of your nervous system.

Sit still in this position for 30 seconds to a minute.

橢法養生

CHAPTER THREE

BUILDING
YOUR CHI

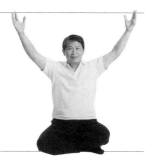

Planning Your Practice

This next stage of your Chi Kung training is called Building Your Chi. There are six fundamental positions that do this. When people start coming to my classes, they often ask if sitting still will really build up their energy. If I give them a long talk about chi, they won't actually have any first-hand experience of it. So, instead, I ask them to try holding the posture and experience the chi for themselves.

Each of the six positions is explained with a series of three photographs. You'll see the posture from the front and side and you'll get a close-up of particularly important details in each position.

You'll find all the details you need for each position on the pages facing the photographs. That way, you get a complete set of instructions for each position. You'll also find the page references for more detailed advice and sample schedules you'll need later on to create your own practice routines. You'll need these suggestions, since eventually you'll be practising these positions, and others presented later in the book, in different combinations.

When you feel confident with the exercises in Gathering your Chi (described on pages 14–33), you will be ready to learn the six fundamental Chi Kung positions that build your chi. Before you begin to practise any of these positions, always do the preliminary practices for Gathering your Chi. Those opening practices are essential for opening and stretching your internal energy pathways and for starting the process of gathering the natural energy that constantly surrounds you.

At the end of this section, after you are introduced to the six positions, there are four closing practices that you should always use to conclude your Chi Kung training. You will find these on pages 76–83.

If you are new to Chi Kung

If this is your first opportunity to learn Chi Kung or if you have not previously tried this particular system, it is important to start with a relaxed attitude. Many new students ask me how long it will take them to become good at Chi Kung. I remind them about the way we help plants and trees grow. It is important that we give them good soil, fresh air and enough water. But if we over-water them or try to make them grow faster by pulling them, it doesn't help. We have to let nature work in its own way.

The same is true for Chi Kung. You already have the good soil you need for your practice: you have a human body. No matter what state of health you are in, your body is remarkable. Its internal energy can be nurtured and strengthened. You have fresh air for your practice: this is literally what you need – make sure the atmosphere around you is not stale. If you can, open a window a little in the room where you do your training. The third thing you need is water: your daily training. Some every day is the secret, not too much, not too little. Don't rush yourself. Just follow the step-by-step approach in this book, taking your time patiently. Like a tree, you will be growing from within.

Here is how you should approach your practice for the first couple of months.

You will get the greatest benefit from Chi Kung practice if you do a little every day. Fifteen minutes daily will make a noticeable difference to your life.

Always begin with the preliminary practices. Then spend up to ten minutes practising the stationary positions to which you are being introduced in this section. Then finish with the concluding practices at the end of this section.

Use the two schedules for Level One and Level Two on the next two pages as the timetable for your practice.

Level One: Training in the first position

The Preliminary Practices	**Essential to begin with these every day**
Extending forward (pages 16–17)	• Extend your arms forward eight times
Side to side (pages 18–19)	• Turn from side to side eight times
Double rubbing (pages 20)	• Rub your knees 12 times
Gathering (pages 26–9)	• Extend 30 seconds to a minute
Sealing (pages 30–3)	• Hands in position 30 seconds to a minute
The Position	**Practice Time**
Lifting	• Start with three minutes on Day One
	• Add a minute every day until you can hold the position for ten minutes
	• Practise holding the position for ten minutes every day for a week
The Concluding Practices	**Essential to end with these everyday**
Pounding the legs and arms (pages 76–7)	Both legs and arms once
Washing the face and neck (pages 78–9)	Once
Circling down (pages 80–1)	Once
Sealing (pages 82–3)	Hands in position 30 seconds to a minute

Level Two: Training in the six positions

The Preliminary Practices	Essential to begin with these every day
Extending forward (pages 16–17) Side to side (pages 18–19) Double rubbing (pages 20–1) Gathering (pages 26–9) Sealing (pages 30–3)	• Extend your arms forward eight times • Turn from side to side eight times • Rub your knees 12 times • Extend 30 seconds to a minute • Hands in position 30 seconds to a minute
The Positions Lifting Holding Expanding Supporting Floating Pressing	**Practice Time** • Always include one minute every day • Add each new position, starting with three minutes on the first day. Then add a minute every day until you can hold the new position for nine minutes • Practise holding the new position for nine minutes every day for a week • Do the same for each position
The Concluding Practices Pounding the legs and arms (pages 76–7) Washing the face and neck (pages 78–9) Circling down (pages 80–1) Sealing (pages 82–3)	**Essential to end with these every day** Both legs and arms once Once Once Hands in position 30 seconds to a minute

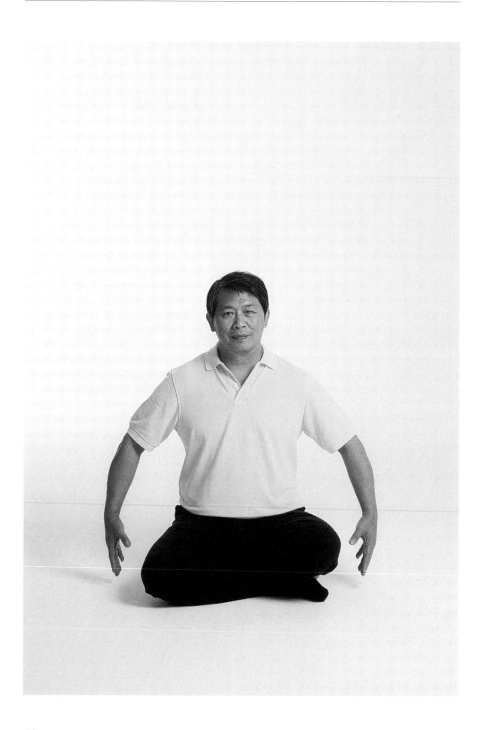

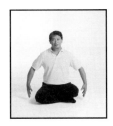 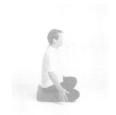 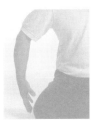

Lifting

This is the first of the six fundamental Chi Kung positions that you are going to learn. After you have completed the preliminary practice of Gathering your Chi *(see pages 26–9),* begin with this position.

Start by sitting comfortably. Your body weight rests on your sitting bones. Your back is naturally upright. You feel your body hanging naturally from the uppermost point on the top of your head.

Let your arms hang loosely by your sides. Relax your shoulders.

Slowly open your elbows outward, away from your body. Then gently raise your elbows so that your forearms and hands begin to move upward beside you.

If you are sitting on the floor, raise your elbows until they lift your hands just clear of the floor. If you are sitting on a low stool or chair, raise your elbows until your wrists clear a line level with the tops of your thighs.

It is extremely important not to hunch your shoulders as you raise your elbows. The movement should be completely relaxed, led from the elbows.

Begin your Chi Kung practice by holding this position for one to five minutes daily.

Breathe naturally.

Follow the detailed advice about this position that follows on pages 42–5.

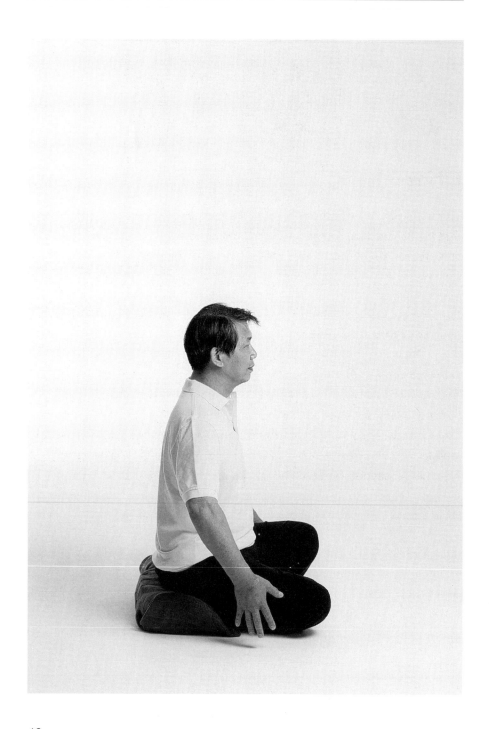

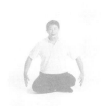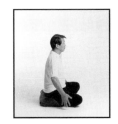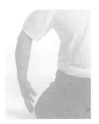

Lifting

When you open your elbows outward in this position, be careful not to pull them backward. As you can see from the photo on the facing page, the shoulders are not drawn backward. The chest remains completely relaxed, just as it was when you were sitting with your arms loosely by your sides.

The forearms slope slightly forward, in the direction of the knees. They do not point straight down to the ground.

There is a subtle inner sense of lifting, from which this position takes its name. You feel as if there were small weights attached to the ends of your fingers. You feel as if you were gently lifting them up. This lift does not come from your shoulders. It comes from your elbows. It does not require you to tense any muscle. There is no external movement. You begin by imagining the action and the inner sensation develops in its own time.

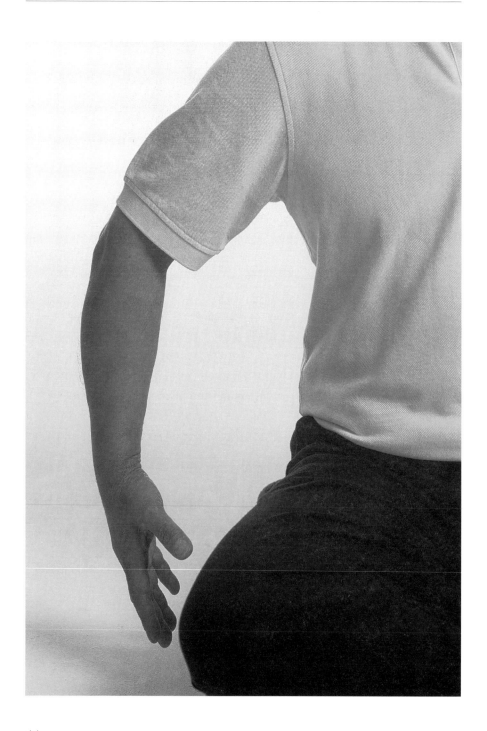

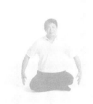 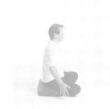 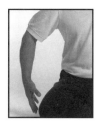

Lifting

You move into this position by opening your elbows outward. This has the effect of creating space under your armpits and between your upper arms and your chest.

This space removes any possible pressure from your arms on your rib cage. It ensures the unrestricted movement of your chest as you breathe.

As you sit in this position, imagine an inflated ball resting in the space under your armpits. Let the weight of your shoulders and upper arms sink into that space, so that you feel you are relaxing into the invisible, resilient support of the inflated ball.

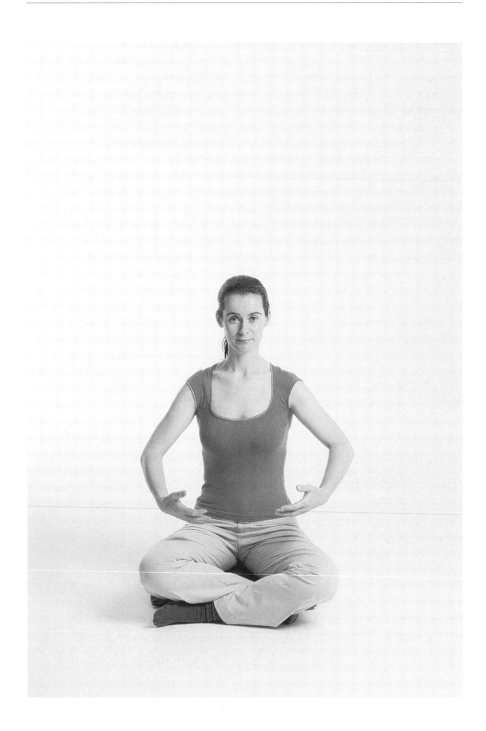

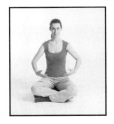 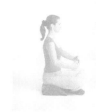 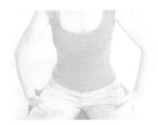

Holding

Sit comfortably, aware of your body weight resting on the floor, stool, support cushion or chair. Straighten your back, but be careful not to tense the muscles in your torso. Feel your bone structure resting naturally in place from the top of your head down to the bottom of your spine.

Let your arms hang loosely by your sides. Relax your shoulders. Slowly open your elbows outward, away from your body.

Then bring your hands in front of your lower abdomen as if gently holding a large ball in front of your belly.

It is extremely important to keep your chest completely relaxed in this position. Do not struggle to hold your arms up with the muscles of your upper torso. Feel that your elbows and shoulders are completely relaxed as you hold the ball in front of your belly.

Breathe naturally.

Follow the detailed advice about this position that follows on pages 48–51.

Try holding this position in accordance with the graduated schedules given on pages 38–9. Once you have completed Level Two of your training, consult the sample schedules on pages 88–9 for advice on developing an advanced daily routine.

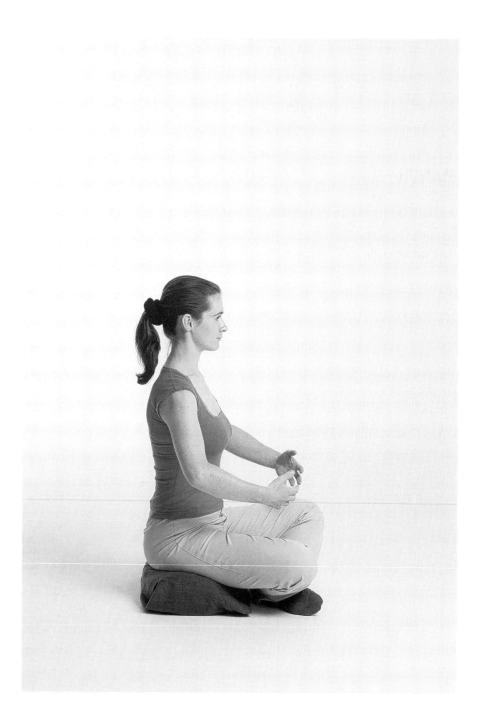

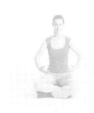
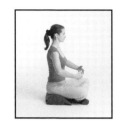
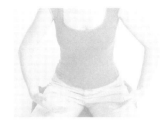

Holding

As you practise holding the imaginary ball in front of your abdomen, be careful not to pull your chest and shoulders backward. This will create strain in your upper body and block the flow of chi.

Although your chest is relaxed, do not slump forward. This will compress your chest and constrict your breathing.

You should have a sense of sitting calmly upright, without strain, with the imaginary ball effortlessly resting between your hands. If you prefer you can imagine that your hands are resting around an expansive belly. You should feel completely relaxed and inwardly happy – in Chinese culture a rotund belly is a sign of wealth and inner power!

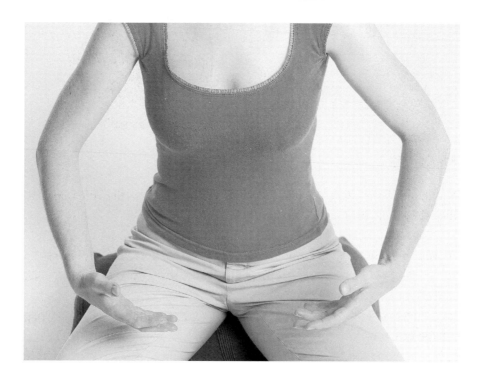

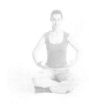
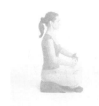
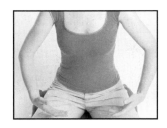

Holding

Your hands hold a large imaginary ball in this position – as they do in most of these Chi Kung postures.

As you imagine your hands holding the ball, your palms naturally develop a soft curve, as if gradually moulding themselves to the surface of the large ball.

Your fingers also are gently curved, just as they would be if you were holding a large beach ball.

There are small spaces between your fingers, which you should hold gently spread apart, as naturally happens when you catch or throw a large ball.

It is this feeling of holding a large ball that gives this position its distinctive inner sensation.

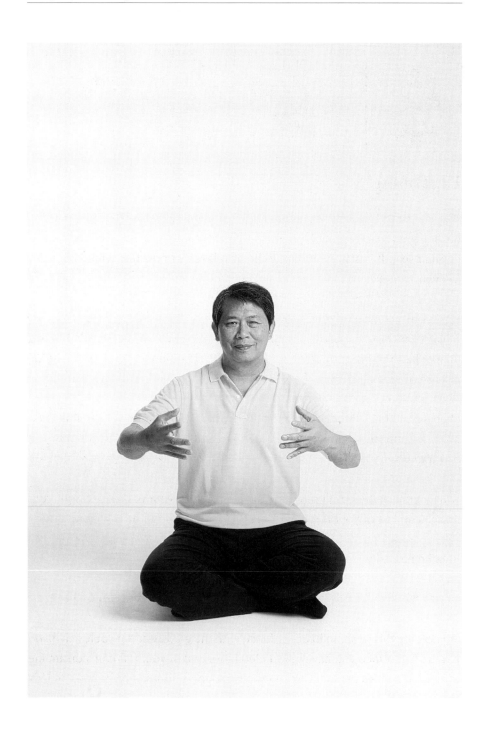

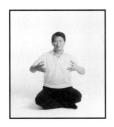 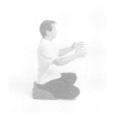 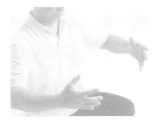

Expanding

Taking a strong, solid seat is especially important in this position. You need to be well grounded – through your contact with the floor, stool, support cushion or chair seat. It is also important to be as relaxed as possible, while maintaining your upright posture.

Start with your hands resting beside your body. As in the previous position, Holding, bring your hands in front of your lower abdomen as if gently holding a large ball in front of your belly. Relax in that position for a moment, getting a sense of the ball between your hands.

Then slowly raise the ball up in front of your chest. Be sure you do this without hunching your shoulders. Only your forearms should move as you raise the ball into position.

You can check the position of your arms by folding your hands in toward your body – the tips of your middle fingers will touch the mid-point of your chest.

Breathe naturally.

Follow the detailed advice about this position that follows on pages 54–7.

Try holding this position in accordance with the graduated schedules given on pages 38–9. Once you have completed Level Two of your training, consult the sample schedules on pages 88–9 for advice on developing an advanced daily routine.

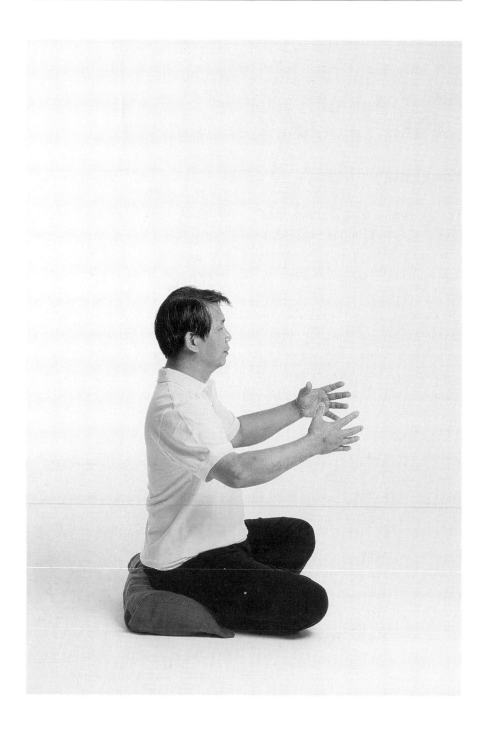

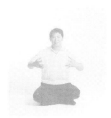 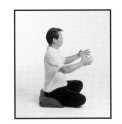 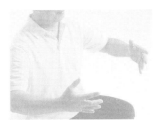

Expanding

Your hands are level with the mid-point of your chest. As you can see, your wrists are slightly higher than your elbows.

To help you relax while holding this position, imagine that there are balloons under each of your armpits. These balloons fill the space under your armpits and support the weight of your upper arm. As you relax into these balloons, you feel a sense of release in your shoulders.

Also imagine that there are balloons supporting your forearms. You feel you are letting all the weight of your forearms sink into these balloons. As you let the balloons take this weight, you feel your chest relaxing.

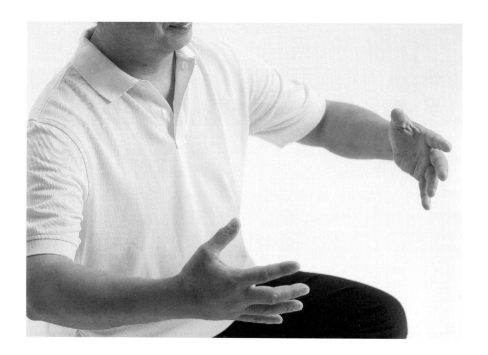

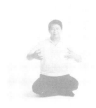 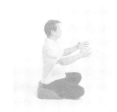 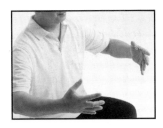

Expanding

When you move your arms into this position, you feel you are lifting a ball between your hands. Once your hands are in place opposite the mid-point of your chest, the sensation changes.

Now you feel that you are holding a large inflated ball inside the circle of your arms. You feel this large ball between your hands, arms and chest.

While you hold the large ball gently in place, it begins to expand as if it was very slowly filling with more air. Your arms and hands remain still, holding the expanding ball. This does not require muscular effort. There is no external movement. It feels more as if you were leaning your arms slightly inward to contain the ball.

As you hold the ball calmly in place, you feel a slight pressure expanding outward through your hands and arms. It is this invisible expansion that gives this position its name.

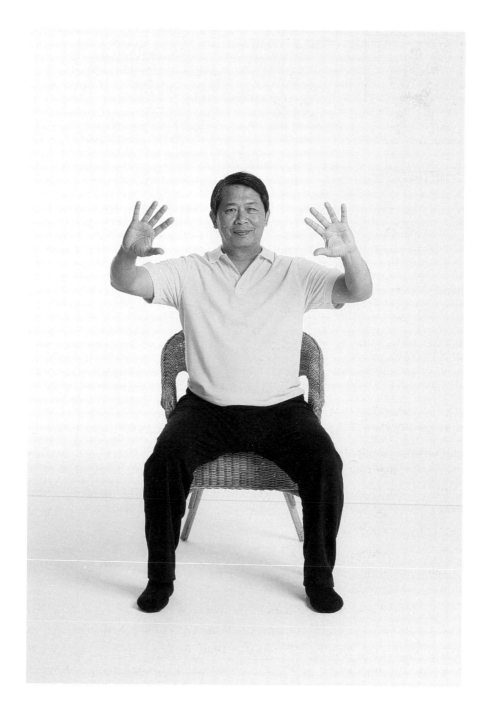

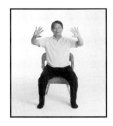 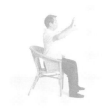 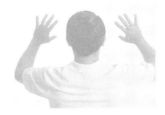

Supporting

As you sit in this position, feel that you are resting on the base of a triangle formed by your two feet and the base of your spine. This triangle feels different when you sit on the floor, low stool, support cushion or chair, but the three main points of contact with earth energy are the same: your two feet and the base of your spine. Establishing a solid base for this position is important, since you will experience higher levels of energy in this more advanced posture.

You begin with your hands resting beside your body. Then bring your hands in front of your belly in the Holding Position. Relax in that position for a moment.

Then slowly raise the ball up in front of your chest, to the Expanding Position. Be sure you do this without hunching your shoulders. Hold that position for a moment. Continue raising the ball until it is level with your face. Then turn the ball outward so that your palms face away from you. Check that your shoulders are relaxed. Do not strain yourself in this position. If you find that it is too powerful for you, slowly lower your arms back to holding the ball in front of your chest or belly.

Breathe naturally.

Follow the detailed advice about this position that follows on pages 60–3. Try holding this position in accordance with the graduated schedules given on pages 38–9. Once you have completed Level Two of your training, consult the sample schedules on pages 88–9 for advice on developing an advanced daily routine.

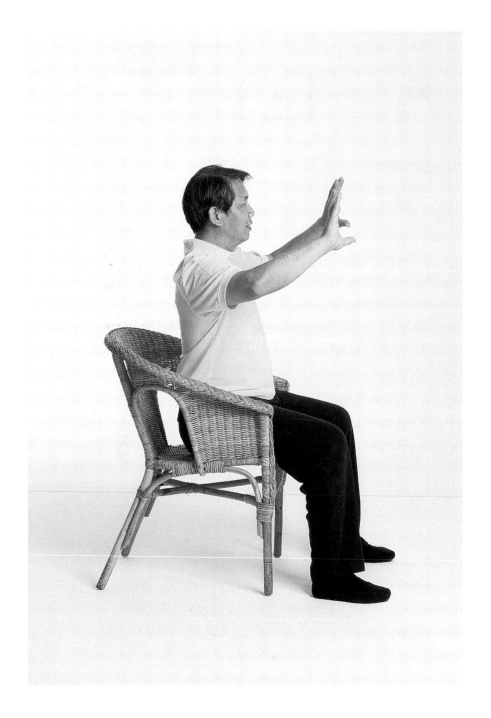

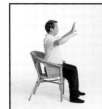
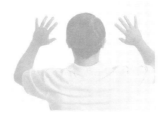

Supporting

Your hands are level with your head. As you can see from the photo, they are not held close to the face but are extended slightly out from your body.

When you move your arms into this position, you may sometimes feel a tendency to lean forward. You can correct this by imagining that there is an elastic cord between the back of your neck and your wrists. There is a subtle sense that you are counterbalancing the pull of your arms with the weight of your upper back. This feeling keeps you upright, without tension.

If you feel pressure or tension in your chest, exhale slowly and allow your shoulders to relax further. Sometimes it helps to imagine that your elbows are extending a little forward, as if creating more space in front of your chest.

If you feel you are straining in this position, open your hands a little outward and lower them slightly.

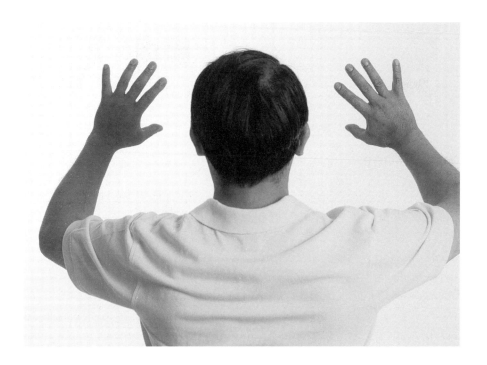

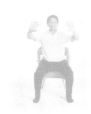 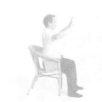 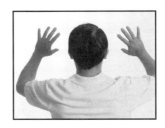

Supporting

Your palms are turned outward, away from your face. They are also turned slightly upward. Imagine that your hands are supporting a large ball in the air. The ball is in front of you, and when you look forward, you can see it in front of you.

The upward turn of your hands is very gentle. Simply rotate your forearms a little so that your palms turn naturally upward a degree or two. There should be no strain in your wrists, and the skin on the backs of your hands and wrists should not form deep creases.

As you hold this position, you feel you are supporting the weight of the ball. This support comes not only from your hands but from the triangle of your entire body, beginning at the base of your sitting posture. This sensation throughout your body is what gives this position its name.

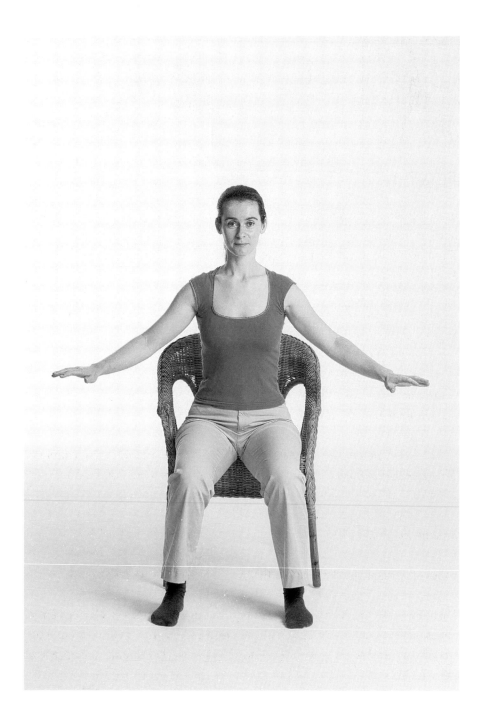

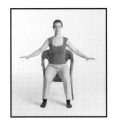 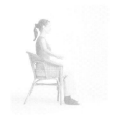 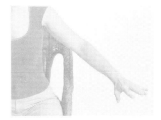

Floating

In China, there are small dolls that are shaped like rounded pyramids. They have a wide, rounded base that makes it impossible to knock them over. Try sitting like this, feeling that you could rock in any direction but remain stable and balanced.

To move into this next position, begin as always with your arms resting loosely by your sides.

Open your elbows outward to open up the space between your ribcage and your upper arms. Then lift your forearms up and out so that they are extended away from your body to each side.

Relax your shoulders and allow the full weight of your arms to rest calmly in the space around them. As in the other Chi Kung positions you have learned, the fingers of both hands are gently spread apart.

Breathe naturally.

Follow the detailed advice about this position that follows on pages 66–9.

Try holding this position in accordance with the graduated schedules given on pages 38–9. Once you have completed Level Two of your training, consult the sample schedules on pages 88–9 for advice on developing an advanced daily routine.

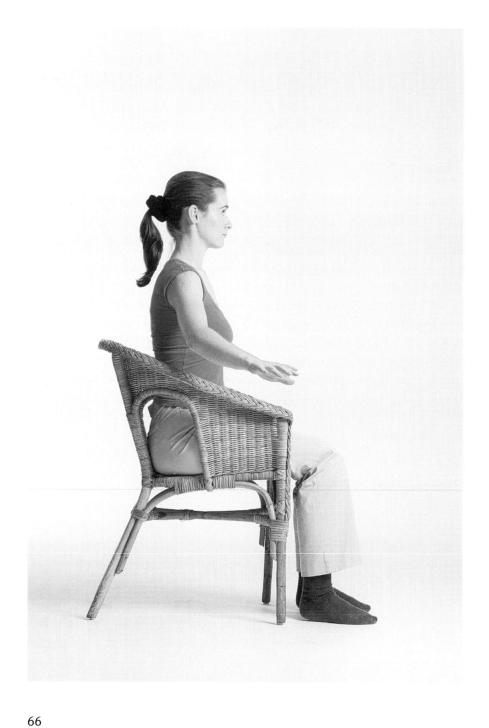

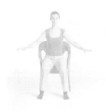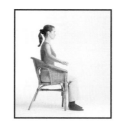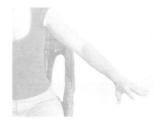

Floating

When you extend your forearms to the side, be careful not to pull your shoulders back. The hands are positioned a little in front of the line of your body. Rather than extended straight out to the sides, your forearms are angled slightly forward.

It is important to keep your shoulders, elbows and wrists relaxed so that each arm forms a gentle curve. There are no sharp angles and no points of tension to block the smooth flow of chi.

Remember the balloons under your armpits, which help support your arms. In addition, you can imagine a strap running around the back of your neck and connecting with your wrists. If you allow the weight of your arms to sink into the strap, you will feel your arms being supported from the point where the strap passes around the back of your neck.

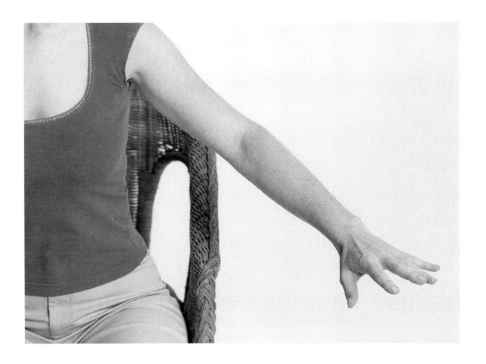

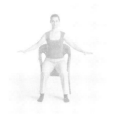 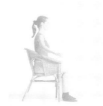 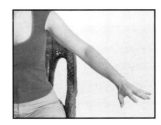

Floating

There is a subtle curve in each wrist. Incline your forearms slightly downward from the elbow, so that your hands are level with your hips. Extend your hands in the same direction as your forearms.

Imagine that there is a balloon under the palm of each hand. These balloons are floating on top of a gently moving stream. Rest the weight of your hands on top of these floating balloons. This naturally creates a soft curve along the palms and fingers of both hands.

In addition to the balloons under your hands, imagine there is one balancing on the back of each hand. This helps you maintain the sensitivity and inner balance in both of your hands.

As you rest your hands on the balloons, you sense the motion of the water and the way the currents affect the balloons. You are careful not to let them drift away, but you allow them to move with the water while remaining in place.

This sensation of your hands and balloons floating on the water together is what gives this position its name.

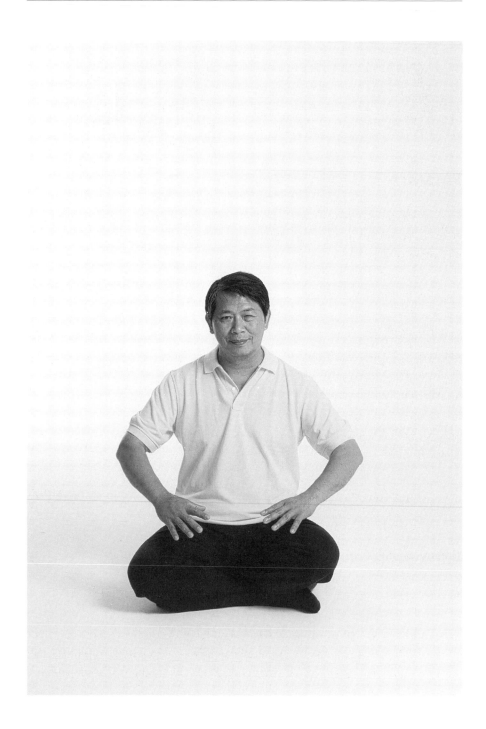

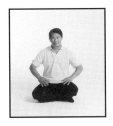 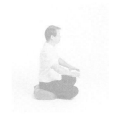 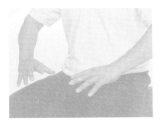

Pressing

Sit like a mountain. The base of the mountain is inseparable from the earth. The great mass of the mountain is concentrated toward its base. At its summit, the mountain is much lighter. It is lofty, completely open to the sun and air.

Begin with your arms hanging effortlessly by your sides.

Slowly bring them in front so that your palms pass just over your knees. They will naturally come together so that the index fingers touch. Then gently open your elbows outward to each side so that a small space opens up between your hands.

Spread the fingers and thumbs of both hands apart so that you can clearly see between them.

Once you have checked the position of your hands, lift your gaze and look forward.

Breathe naturally.

Follow the detailed advice about this position that follows on pages 72–5.

Try holding this position in accordance with the graduated schedules given on pages 38–9. Once you have completed Level Two of your training, consult the sample schedules on pages 88–9 for advice on developing an advanced daily routine.

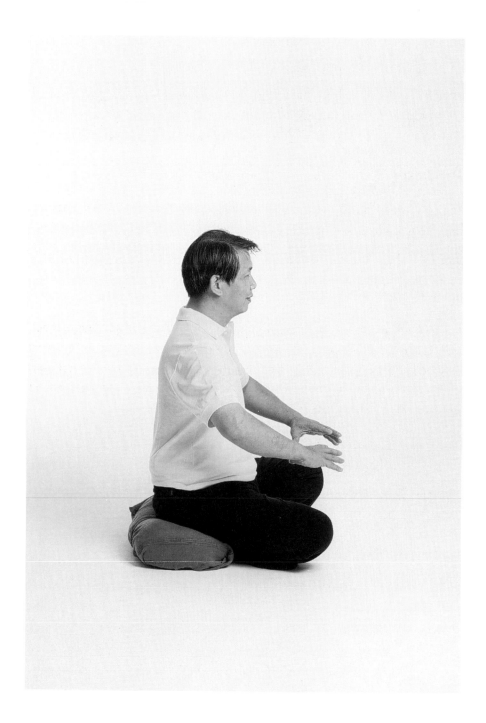

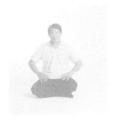 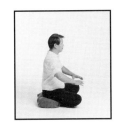 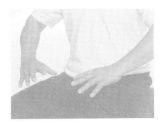

Pressing

Your elbows are slightly in front of the midline of your body. This enables your chest to remain relaxed. You can feel a gentle curve running from your upper spine along your shoulder-blades and out to your elbows.

Your forearms slope very slightly downward from your elbows.

You feel as if you are sitting in the water at the edge of the sea, pressing a beach ball down in the waves. This takes your attention to your palms. At the same time, to keep the ball steady in the waves, you have to exert a little effort from the base of your spine. The feeling produced by your palms and spine as you press on the beach ball is what gives this position its name.

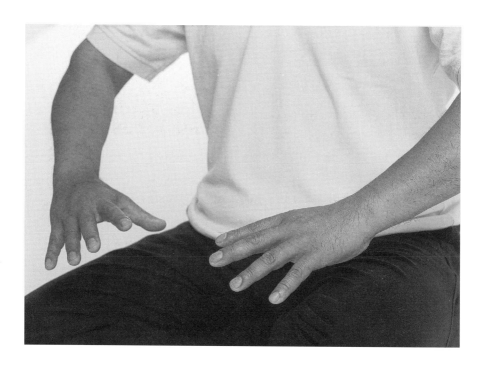

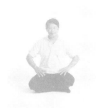 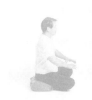 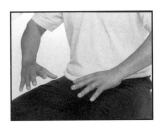

Pressing

If you look down at your hands, you will see that they form a triangle in space. Your two thumbs point toward each other, separated by a small space roughly equivalent to the length of another thumb. The line of your thumbs is the base of the triangle.

The other two lines of the triangle are formed by the middle fingers of each hand. If they extended forward, they would meet, forming the apex of the triangle. You can visualize a small sphere held lightly in the space created by your thumbs and forefingers.

You can see a second triangle as you look down. This is the larger triangle formed by your chest, elbows and hands.

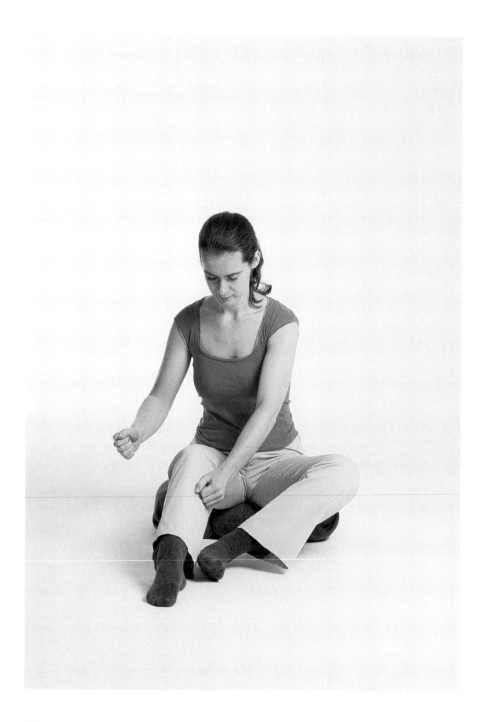

Pounding the legs and arms

At the end of your Chi Kung practice, it is always important to conclude properly. You need to release any tension, relax your nervous system and seal the energy you have generated. Please make a special point of always concluding with the four practices you see here and on the pages that follow.

First, we begin with pounding the legs and arms. This practice is known in Chinese as 'Do Yin'. It stimulates circulation and encourages the flow of blood to the heart.

If you have been sitting with your legs crossed, unfold your legs one at a time.

Fold your hands into loose fists and, taking one leg at a time, begin gently pounding both fists against each leg. Start right down at the ankle and work your way up the leg, making rapid little taps all over the surface of the leg.

Then pound your way up the other leg.

Next come the arms. You won't be able to use both fists on each arm. Just use your right fist to pound all over your left arm, working from the wrist up to the shoulder. Then do the same with your left fist all the way up your right arm.

The pounding action is brisk and vigorous, but not so hard as to cause pain.

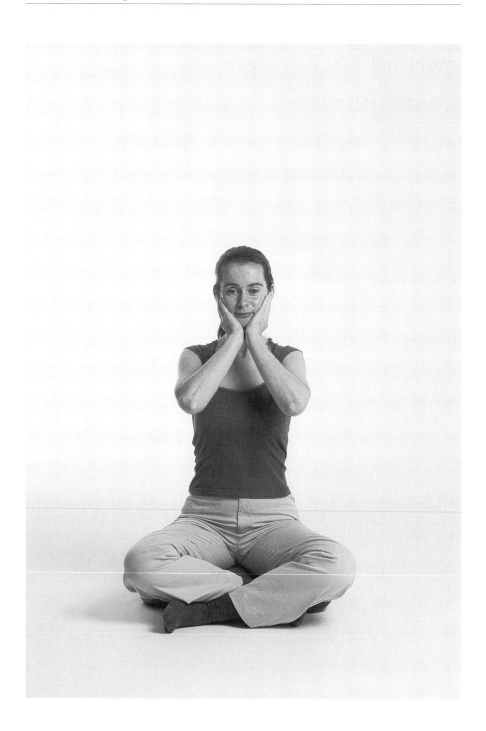

Washing the face and neck

This chi massage is wonderful for releasing tension in the face and neck. It helps to relax the entire nervous system. It is also draws chi right out to the surface of your face and, with regular practice, it gives your skin a noticeable glow, over time.

Place your palms together and then rub them vigorously until you feel both your palms and fingers getting warm.

Then rub your palms all over your face, as if you were giving yourself a good wash. Be sure to include the entire area of your eyes.

Then take your hands to the back of your neck and give yourself a good rub there with both palms.

Finish by holding your hands still on your neck. Relax your arms and let your neck feel the weight of your arms resting on it. You can lock your fingers together while holding your hands against the back of your neck. Or you can place your right hand against the back of your neck and rest your left hand on top of it.

Rest your hands on your neck for a moment, feeling the gentle pressure. Then lower your hands and relax.

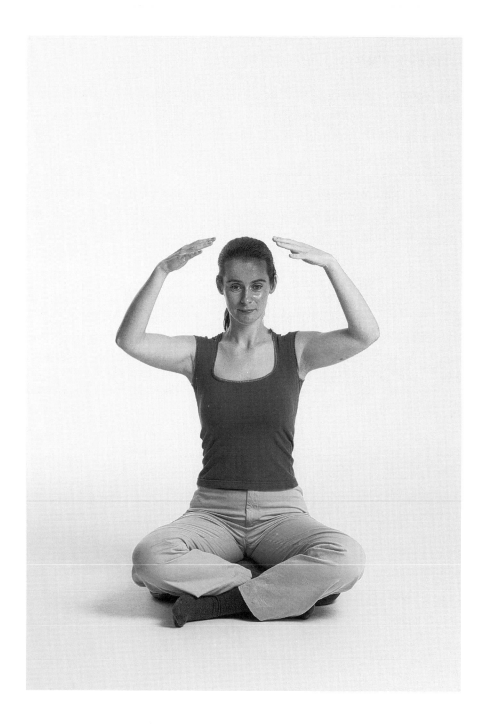

Circling down

This concluding movement directs your energy downward toward your abdomen, where the all-important chi reservoir in your Tan Tien is located. Always do this practice at the end of your session.

Start with your arms out to the side, your palms turned upward. Slowly raise both arms outward and upward in two large arcs circling up beside your body. Your hands meet above the level of your head, slightly away from the front line of your body. There should be a space of about one palm between them.

Breathe in as your arms circle up.

Then slowly press your hands down in front of you until they come to rest opposite your navel. You feel you are pressing a large ball down into water. This makes the movement slow and deliberate, with your attention on your palms as they carefully press the ball down into the water.

Breathe out as your arms press down.

Keep your hands in position in front of your navel, your palms facing downward, for a moment. Then lower them to your sides and relax.

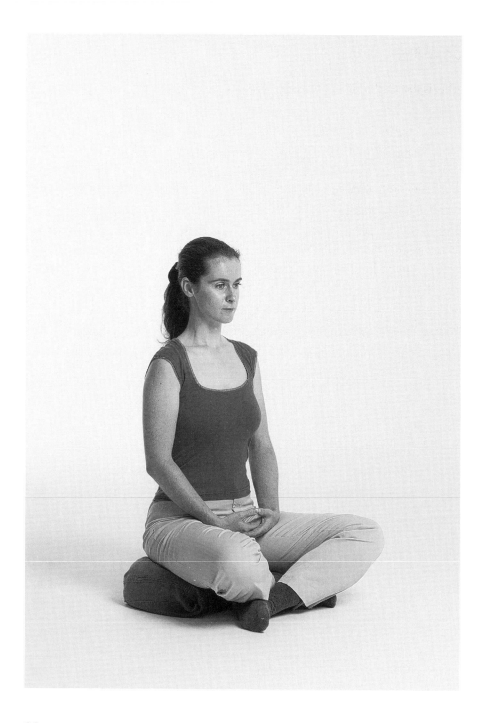

Sealing

This is the final moment of your Chi Kung practice.

Bring your hands together in your lap. Your palms are turned upward. Your right hand rests on top of your left. The tips of your thumbs lightly touch each other.

Let your chest, arms and shoulders relax fully, while your torso, neck and head remain lightly upright.

Imagine the crystal sphere resting in the cradle of your hands in your lap. Its radiant energy is naturally absorbed into the reservoir of your Tan Tien and is quietly sealed into your abdomen, ready for use at any time.

Rest in this position for 30 seconds to a minute.

These are the characters for
'Shih Li' – power testing

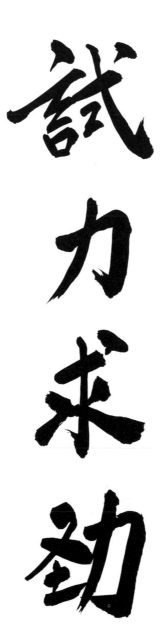

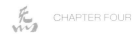

CHAPTER FOUR

GUIDING
YOUR CHI

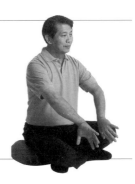

Planning Your Practice

The time you have spent working with the preliminary Chi Kung practices, followed by gathering and building your chi, has prepared you for the next stage of your training.

Now you are ready to move on to more subtle movements. Sometimes people ask me what makes these simple movements different from normal muscle work. The difference is hidden inside the body. The external movement triggers the unseen internal movement of your chi. If you follow the instructions carefully, you'll be able to feel the difference. These small movements are like the little pilot boats that guide large ships through a harbour. Like tea leaves, they are tiny, but they transform water into a cup of tea.

You can do these movements either sitting or standing. But at this stage, in order to ensure that you build up your Chi Kung training properly, please start by doing your training sitting down. You'll be adding the movements step by step to the daily Chi Kung practice you have already established at the end of Level Two.

Once a week try adding a session of Guiding your Chi. Begin with the first movement, Lifting. (The same name is used for this movement as for the first position you have already learned, since the movement is an extension of that position.) The structured schedule for this training is shown in the chart for Level Three on the facing page.

After training in Level Three once a week for a month, you'll be ready to progress to Level Four.

Start by carrying out each movement 36 times, as indicated on the following pages. Once you have completed Level Four, you can progress to a more advanced stage of this training. Feel you are building up the internal pressure of the movement a little with each of the 36 breaths. Relax a bit between each breath as you work up to a maximum pressure on the 36th outbreath.

This type of training is different to ordinary exercise. You are training your energy, not your muscles. The approach is different and the feeling is different. For example, there is no point is trying to get through these movements quickly. In this system, you are not going to get extra benefit if you push yourself beyond the limits of endurance or complete the full set of movements faster and faster every day. The movements are meant to be done carefully and slowly.

The feeling you have when doing these movements is one of careful attention. Of course your mind may wander, but when it does, return to what you are doing. Try to be aware of the entire movement, not just the beginning and ending. No matter how small the movement is, let your mind rest on it fully. Try to enter into the sensation of each movement. Feel your entire hand from the wrist right through to your fingertips. One way to do this is to imagine that you are practising in a huge tub of heavy oil. As you move your hands and arms, you feel every inch of your skin and a sense of the fullness of your limbs as they move through the slight resistance of the oil.

However, make sure you don't tense up or become too serious about this. The movements should be calm and relaxed. In the beginning a lot of my students worry too much about getting everything right and so are unable to release their inner tension. I encourage them not to frown. In fact, a gentle smile is the perfect companion for your practice.

Level Three: Training in the first movement of Guiding your Chi

The Preliminary Practices	**Essential to begin with these every day**
Extending forward (pages 16–17) Side to side (pages 18–19) Double rubbing (pages 20–21) Gathering (pages 26–29) Sealing (pages 30–33)	• Extend your arms forward eight times • Turn from side to side eight times • Rub your knees 12 times • Extend your arms 30 seconds to a minute • Hands in position 30 seconds to a minute
The Positions Lifting Another position	**Practice Time** Always begin with one minute Add five minutes of holding any other position
The First Movement Lifting	**Practice Time** 36 times (once a week over one month)
The Concluding Practices	**Essential to end with these every day**
Pounding the legs and arms (pages 76–7) Washing the face and neck (pages 78–9) Circling down (pages 80–81) Sealing (pages 82–83)	Both legs and arms once Once Once Hands in position 30 seconds to a minute

Level Four: Training in the six movements of Guiding your Chi

The Preliminary Practices	Essential to begin with these every day
Extending forward (pages 16–17) Side to side (pages 18–19) Double rubbing (pages 20–21) Gathering (pages 26–29) Sealing (pages 30–33)	• Extend your arms forward eight times • Turn from side to side eight times • Rub your knees 12 times • Extend your arms 30 seconds to a minute • Hands in position 30 seconds to a minute
The Positions Lifting Another position	**Practice Time** Always begin with one minute Add five minutes of holding any other position
The Six Movements Lifting Holding Expanding Supporting Floating Pressing	**Practice Time** Practise each movement once a week. Each time do the movement 36 times. Train in each movement once a week for a month. Then progress to the next movement. (Level Five counts as the first of these.)
The Concluding Practices Pounding the legs and arms (pages 76–77) Washing the face and neck (pages 78–79) Circling down (pages 80–81) Sealing (pages 82–83)	**Essential to end with these every day** Both legs and arms once Once Once Hands in position 30 seconds to a minute

Lifting

This movement guides your chi upward and downward throughout your upper body, strengthening its circulation throughout your vital organs. It not a hurried movement and is graceful in its ascending and descending motion. It feels like the constant rise and fall of waves. At the end of the sequence shown in these pictures, gracefully return to the starting position and repeat the movement 36 times.

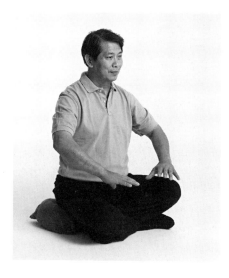 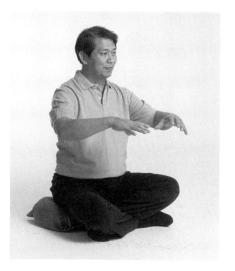

1. Begin by sitting with your hands in front of your body, level with your belly. Your palms and fingers curve slightly downward, as if holding a medium-sized ball. Breathe in.

2. Slowly raise your arms. The backs of your wrists lead the movement. Your palms curve slightly as if lifting a ball. You feel you are lifting a weight attached to your wrists. Breathe out as your hands come up.

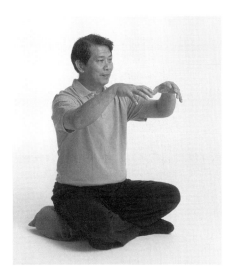

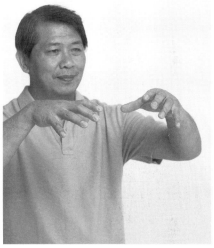

3. Raise your arms until your hands are level with your head. Keep your shoulders and chest completely relaxed.

4. Feel as if your fingertips are connected by invisible elastic to the Tan Tien inside your abdomen. As you lift your hands, feel your Tan Tien being stretched and an inner sense of your whole body pressing downward. You may experience a similar sensation at the Hui Yin point between your legs. You lower your hands to begin the movement again, as if pressing the invisible ball into water while breathing in.

Holding

This movement guides your chi diagonally inward to your Tan Tien, the principal energy reservoir of your system. Although the fourth and final instruction is to press your palms diagonally downward, away from your belly, you do this internally, keeping your hands still. At the end of the sequence shown in these pictures, gracefully return to the starting position and repeat the movement 36 times.

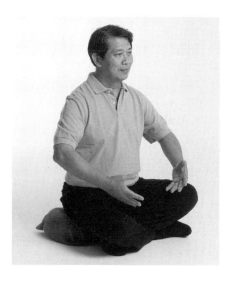 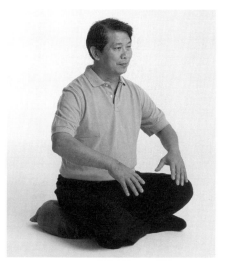

1. Begin by sitting in the second position, Holding. Sit naturally upright. Hold your arms in front of you, as if holding the large inflated ball in front of your belly. Relax your chest. The weight of your upper body is supported by imaginary balloons under your armpits. Sit still in that posture for a moment.

2. Rotate your forearms inward so that the thumbs of both hands start to make a small arc toward each other. Breathe in as you rotate your forearms. Keep your chest and shoulders relaxed.

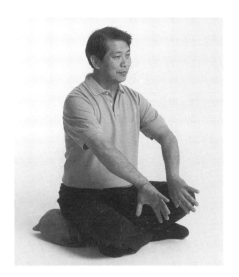

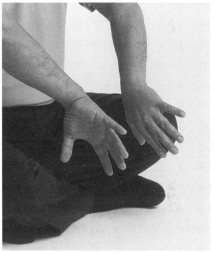

3. Complete the inward rotation of your forearms so that the backs of both hands face each other. Point your fingers diagonally downward and rotate your palms outward. When you look down you clearly see the backs of your hands.

4. Look forward. Keeping your hands still, press both palms diagonally downward and breathe out. To balance the downward twist of your arms, feel as if strong elastic were gently expanding between your wrists and the back of your neck. Your fingertips form an invisible, expanding triangle in front of your Tan Tien.

Expanding

This movement guides your chi horizontally throughout your upper body, strengthening the energy in your heart and lungs. Like pulsing movements of those vital organs, try to make the movement constant and rhythmic. At the end of the sequence shown in these pictures, gracefully return to the starting position and repeat the movement 36 times.

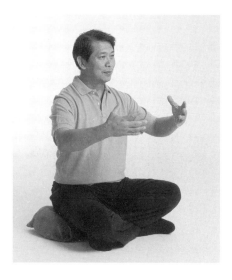 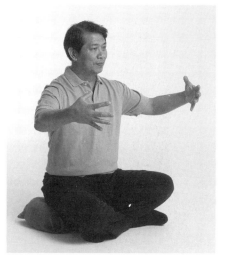

1. Begin by sitting in the third position, Expanding. Sit up holding the imaginary ball between your chest and your arms. Your wrists are slightly higher than your elbows. The weight of your arms is supported by the invisible balloons under your upper arms and forearm. Relax, maintaining your upright posture for a moment.

2. Slowly move both your arms away from each other, leading the movement with the backs of your wrists, until your fingers are about shoulder-width apart. Breathe in as your hands move outward. Keep your chest and shoulders relaxed.

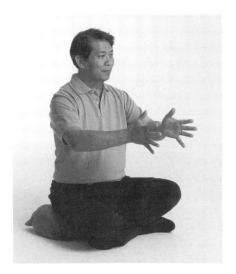

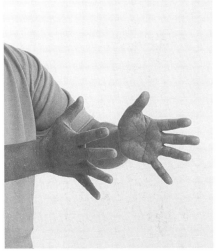

3. Then slowly move your arms in toward each other, leading the movement with the palms of your hands. Breathe out as your hands move inward.

4. This movement is similar to playing an accordion. Look forward. Imagine that you are pulling the accordion as you open your hands, and that you are gently pressing on it as you bring your palms back in toward each other. As you practise, you sense an invisible strap around your neck, supporting the weight of the accordion between your hands.

Supporting

This movement guides your chi diagonally upward and outward, connecting with the energy of the heavens. Don't worry about your energy flying away. You will feel the inner movement of your chi as it naturally moves downward into the reservoir of your Tan Tien. At the end of the sequence shown in these pictures, gracefully return to the starting position and repeat the movement 36 times.

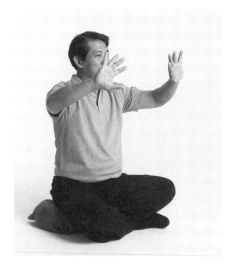 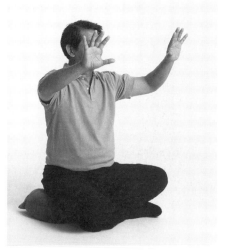

1. Begin by sitting in the fourth position. Turn your hands outward, away from your face, as if supporting a large ball. Completely relax your shoulders and chest. The weight of your upper body is supported by imaginary balloons under your armpits. Stabilize in that posture for a moment. Breathe in.

2. Begin to extend your arms so that your hands are pushed upward and outward toward the upper left and right diagonals. Breathe out as your arms start to extend. Keep your chest and shoulders relaxed.

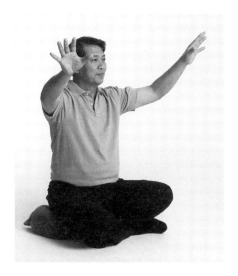

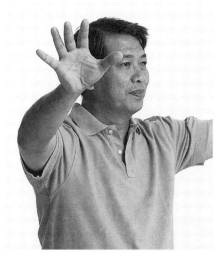

3. Complete the outward and upward extension by spreading your finger and thumbs slightly more apart. You feel as if your hands were like two fans opening outward and unfolding. You feel your energy expanding outward through your fingers, but remain relaxed. Your shoulders, elbows and wrists do not stiffen.

4. Look forward. As your arms and hands extend upward and outward, complete the expansion in the opposite direction using the back of your neck and shoulders. It is as if you were stretching a circle of strong elastic looped around your hands and upper body. Then bring your arms back to the starting position as you breathe in.

Floating

This movement guides your chi forward and backward. You'll feel how calming and deeply relaxing this is. The action is smooth and continuous, like a pendulum. Repeat the full backward and forward movement 36 times.

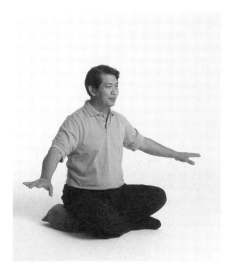 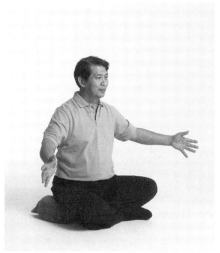

1. Begin by sitting in the fifth position, Floating. Sit up, feeling relaxed. Your hands are extended out to the sides, with your palms facing downward. Be careful not to pull your shoulders and chest back. Your hands are a little in front of the line of your body. Imagine you are sitting comfortably in a swimming pool. Breathe in.

2. Slowly start to move both your arms forward, rotating your hands so that your palms face forward. Breathe out as your hands turn and start to move forward. Keep your chest and shoulders relaxed.

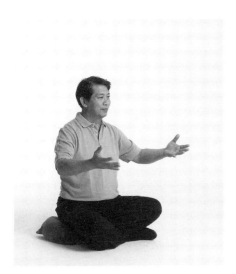 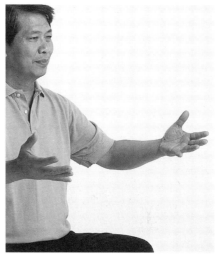

3. As you continue the forward motion, your forearms sweep upward a little. Imagine you are playing in the pool, gently sweeping your hands forward through the water.

4. Look forward. At the end of the forward sweep, relax. Let the backs of your hands trail back down through the water to rest again by your sides. As your hands move back into their original position, breathe in. As you make this delightful movement, you will notice corresponding inner swaying within your Tan Tien.

Pressing

This movement guides your Chi down to the base of your abdomen and connects it with the energy of the earth. Although the fourth and final instruction is to press your palms downward, you do this internally, keeping your hands still. At the end of the sequence shown in these pictures, gracefully return to the starting position and repeat the movement 36 times.

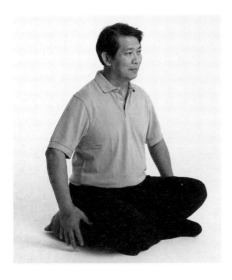 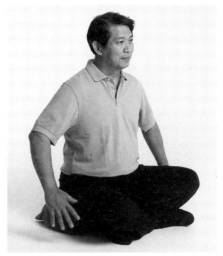

1. Begin by sitting with your back upright. Hold your arms by your sides, away from your body. Relax your shoulders and upper arms into the imaginary balloons under your armpits. Stabilize yourself, sitting calmly in that posture for a moment.

2. Rotate your wrists inward so that the thumbs of both hands start to make a small arc toward your thighs. Breathe in as you rotate your wrists into position. Keep your chest and shoulders relaxed.

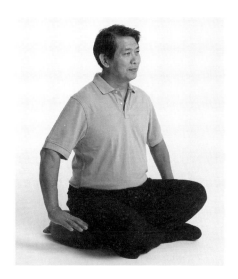

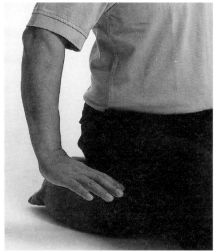

3. Complete the inward rotation of your hands so that the fingers of both hands point straight ahead and the palms face downward. Your hands are now parallel with the ground. When you look down you see the backs of your hands.

4. Look forward. Keeping you hands still, press down both palms downward and breathe out. Imagine your palms are internally connected by elastic to the back of your neck and to your Tan Tien. There is a reaction to the downward pressure of your hands. You feel you are being subtly straightened from within.

*These are the characters for
'Yi Jin Ching' – tendon changing,
the internal strengthening of the
muscles, tendons and bones.*

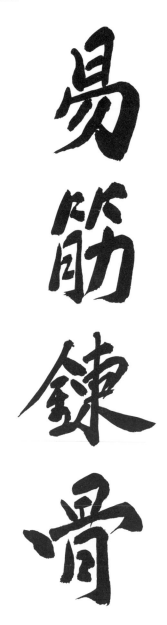

CHAPTER FIVE

INCREASING
YOUR CHI

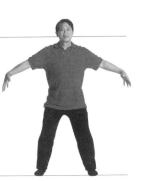

Planning for Practice

Now that you have spent some time learning the Chi Kung practices that gather, build and guide your chi, you can move on to more advanced positions that increase it.

You'll find these advanced positions greatly increase the flow of chi throughout your system, so it is all the more important that you strengthen yourself internally first. It's just the same as it is with electricity: we need strong cables to carry high levels of electric power. That is why I advise my students to build up their daily practice gradually. You can do the same thing by following the order of daily practice set out in the charts at the beginning of each section of this book. Before starting the training in this section, do your best to complete each of the four levels of training presented on pages 38–9 and 88–9.

There's a set of three photographs showing each of the advanced positions in this section. They show you the posture from the front and side and also give you a close-up of a particularly important detail of the position. You'll find all the details you need for each position on the pages facing the photographs.

You can do these advanced positions either sitting or standing. But to begin with, I recommend you do them sitting. As you can see from the training schedule for Level Five on the facing page, you'll be starting and finishing with the Preliminary and Concluding Practices with which you are already familiar.

When you have finished your training in these positions, gently fold your hands over your abdomen. Place your right hand against your belly and hold your left hand over it. Sit or stand still, holding your hands comfortably in place to lock your chi into your Tan Tien. Breathe naturally. This is an advanced practice for sealing your energy, appropriate for this level of training.

Once a week, I recommend you try these positions while standing. That will take you to Level Six. Before starting, please pay careful attention to the explanation for the Holding Posture on pages 120–5. The Preliminary and Concluding Practices change when you do standing Chi Kung. They are different to the ones you have already learned. Follow the instructions carefully and always begin and conclude your Chi Kung training with these new practices. The structured schedule for this training is shown in the chart for Level Six.

Since the standing practice of Chi Kung increases the flow of Chi in your system to higher levels, you may experience new sensations. These vary from person to person. For example, different sides of your body may feel different. One hand may feel cold while the other one is hot. Your skin may tingle. You might sweat a lot. Your digestive system may become active, producing gurgles and gas. You might find old aches and pains coming back for a while. Some people shake while standing. All these sensations, including emotional effects, are completely normal. Your internal energy is rebalancing. Like a river in spring, it is following freely after being blocked up in winter.

When you use the charts on the next two pages, you will see that they refer to the preliminary and concluding practices. By now, you should be thoroughly familiar with these exercises and know them by heart. If you are unsure what to do, just check back with the charts for Levels One to Four.

Once you are familiar with the practices given in Level Five, you can gradually start training in the standing positions before starting Level Six. The way to do this is to add a few minutes of standing practice once a week. On that day, instead of your usual practice of Level Five, follow the instructions for Level Six. Then, for the rest of the week, return to your Level Five practice. This way you will make a gradual transition to Level Six without straining yourself.

Level Five: Training in the advanced positions while sitting

The Preliminary Practices *(pages 14–33)*	Essential to begin with these every day
The six advanced positions Lifting (pages 114–19) Holding (pages 120–5) Expanding (pages 126–31) Supporting (pages 127–37) Floating (pages 140–3) Pressing (pages 144–9)	• Start with three minutes on Day One and Two • Add a minute every two days until you can hold the position for ten minutes • Practise holding the position for ten minutes every day for two weeks • Thereafter include one minute of this position before training in the next five • Start with three minutes of each new position • Add a minute of each new position every two days until you can hold the new position for nine minutes • Practise holding the new position for nine minutes every day for two weeks • Do the same for each position
The Concluding Practices *(pages 90–101)* Weekly standing practice	Essential to end with these every day Once a week, insert a day of standing practice as recommended in the chart below

Level Six: Training in the advanced positions while standing

The Preliminary Practices Strengthening the knees (pages 108–9) Rotating the hips (pages 110–11) Relaxing the shoulders (pages 112–13)	**Essential to begin with these every day** • 12 rotations each direction • 12 rotations each direction • 12 arm circles
Original Position Lifting (pages 40–5) **The Six Advanced Positions** Lifting (pages 114–19) Holding (pages 120–5) Expanding (pages 126–31) Supporting (pages 127–37) Floating (pages 140–3) Pressing (pages 144–9)	**Practice Time** • One minute • Start with three minutes the first week. • Add a minute each week until you can stand in the position for ten minutes. • Stand in the position for ten minutes once a week for six weeks. Thereafter include one minute standing in this position before training in the next five. • Add a minute of each new position each week until you are holding the new position for eight minutes. • Stand in each new position for eight minutes once a week for eight weeks • Do the same for each position
The Concluding Practices Hitting the drum (pages 150–1) Shaking hands and feet (pages 152–3) Circling down and sealing (pages 154–5)	**Essential to end with these every day** 12 hits on the drum 30 seconds to a minute Hands in position 30 seconds to a minute

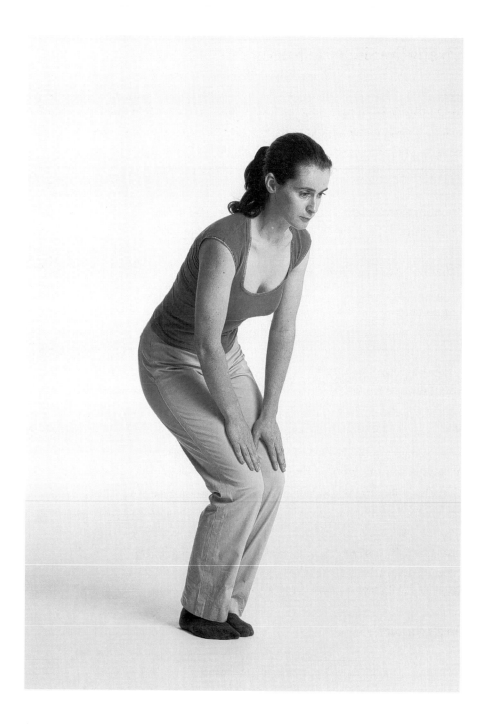

Strengthening the knees

In the earlier sections of this book, you learned a set of preliminary practices that are essential before doing Chi Kung training in a sitting position. Since this section concentrates on the standing practice of Chi Kung, you'll need to do a different set of Preliminary Practices. Always begin with these.

This movement helps to strengthen and relax your entire lower body. It releases tension in all the joints from the hips down to the ankles.

Stand with your feet together.

Bend your knees a little.

Slide your hands down your thighs until your hands come to rest just above your kneecaps. Be careful not to lean too far forward or put any pressure on your legs.

Relax your lower back.

Your head is in line with your torso. Don't stare straight down at your feet, or straight ahead. Let your gaze naturally settle on a space about 2 m (6 ft) in front of you on the ground.

Slowly rotate your knees 12 times to the left and 12 times to the right.

Try to keep the soles of your feet flat on the ground.

Breathe naturally.

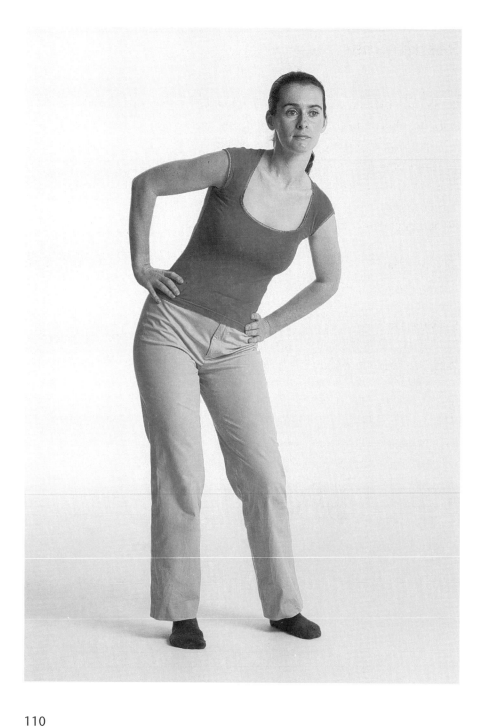

Rotating the hips

If you want to build your chi up to its highest level, you really need a relaxed, powerful abdomen. Many people have a very tense belly, which is like putting a big lock on the door to their main reservoir of chi. So it is extremely important to release tension in the belly before doing advanced Chi Kung practice. This movement helps relax the entire musculature of the middle body.

Stand upright with your feet shoulder-width apart.

Rest your hands on your hips. Relax your shoulders by letting the full weight of your arms be supported by the connection of your hands and hips.

Slowly rotate your hips 12 times to the left and 12 times to the right.

Keep your head gently upright as you make this gentle movement.

Let your abdomen soften and your lower back relax.

Breathe naturally.

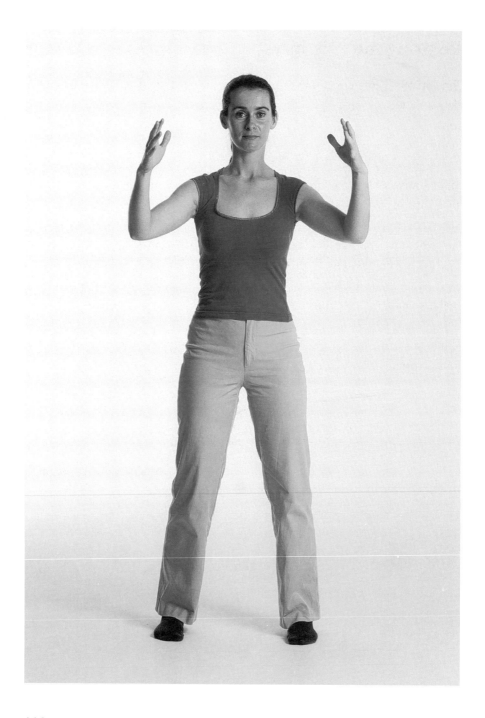

Relaxing the shoulders

Tension often rises upward in our bodies, causing stiffness in the chest, shoulders and neck. These arm circles help relax the entire upper torso.

Stand comfortably with your feet shoulder-width apart.

Slowly raise your arms as if lifting a large ball. Be careful not to hunch your shoulders or stiffen your arms. Breathe in with the upward movement.

Turn your arms outward and gently lower them back to start again. Breathe out as your arms circle downward.

Make at least 12 slow complete circles with your arms.

When you have finished, let your arms rest naturally at your sides. Stand still for a moment, breathing naturally.

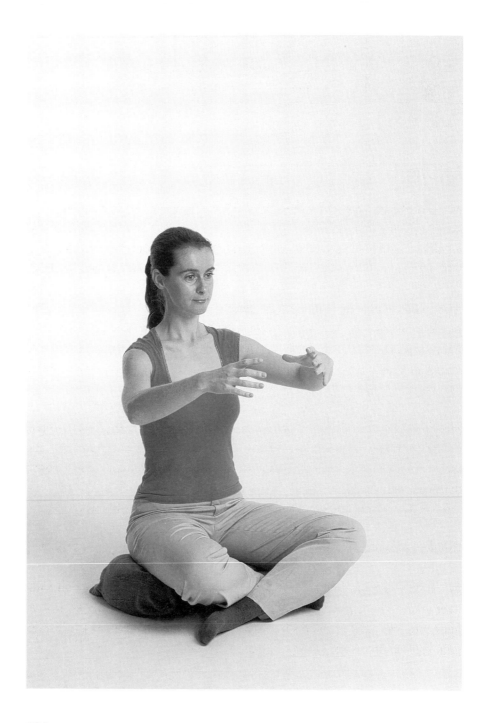

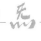

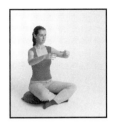 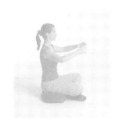 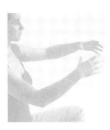

Lifting

Many of the photographs in this section show how to do the position while standing rather than sitting. You can do them either way. Your chi will increase whether you hold the positions while standing or sitting. Once you try them you will find that holding the positions while standing is definitely more powerful.

If you choose to hold these advanced positions while sitting, as in this example, it is all the more important to establish a sold, stable base as the ground for your practice. Feel yourself connecting with the earth as you sit, and the weight of your body resting firmly on your sitting bones. Your upper body, neck and head feel light and free from tension.

Start with your hands in the position, Pressing, on pages 70–5, then raise your hands until they are level with your shoulders. In the original position, your wrists are lower than your elbows. In this advanced position, they are higher than your elbows. As you hold your hands in this higher position, pay particular attention to relaxing your chest, shoulders and neck. Breathe naturally.

Follow the detailed advice about this position that follows on pages 116–19.

When you have finished your training in this position, gently fold your hands over your abdomen. Place your right hand against your belly and hold your left hand over it. Sit or stand still, holding your hands comfortably in place to lock your chi into your Tan Tien. Breathe naturally.

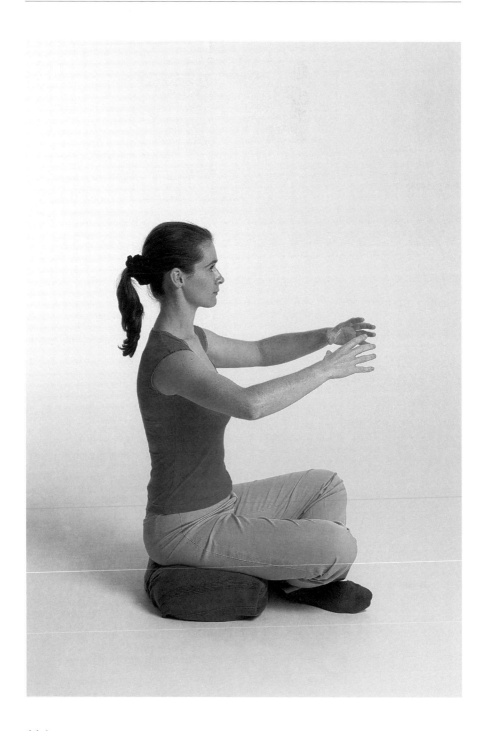

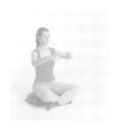
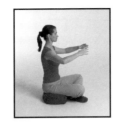
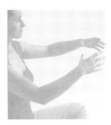

Lifting

The simplest way to move into this posture is to begin in the original Pressing Position described on pages 70–5.

In the original position your hands rest in the space in front of your abdomen, forming an open triangle with your palms facing downward.

Now imagine that there is an invisible cord attached to the central point on the back of each hand. Imagine that your hands and arms are pulled up by the cords attached to these points.

Your hands are pulled up until the backs of your hands are level with your shoulders.

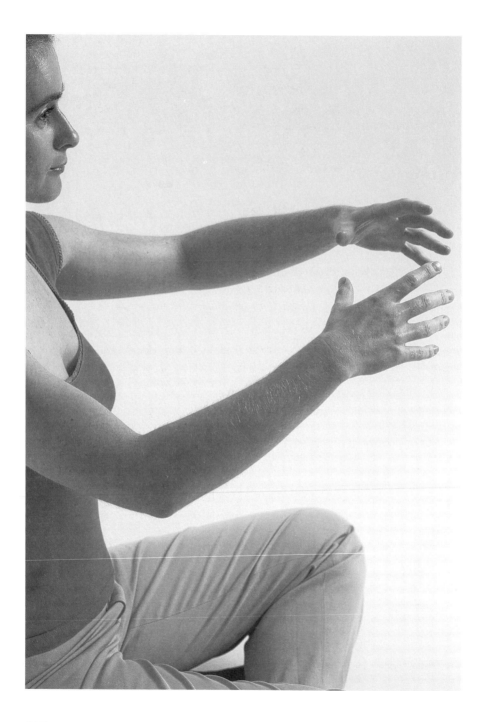

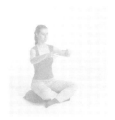 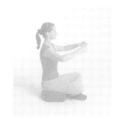 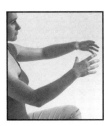

Lifting

In this advanced position the curve of your palms and fingers is more pronounced than before. You feel as if each hand is holding a medium-sized ball, about the size of a grapefruit. Your palms and fingers hold the balls from above. This naturally deepens the pocket of your palms, and your fingers keep the balls in place.

Once your hands are in position, relax them to release any unnecessary strain.

From time to time, as you hold this position, check that your chest, shoulders and neck are relaxed.

You begin to feel that you are continuously lifting the two invisible balls under your palms. The effort involved in holding your arms up slowly ebbs away as you feel the constant lifting sensation in your hands.

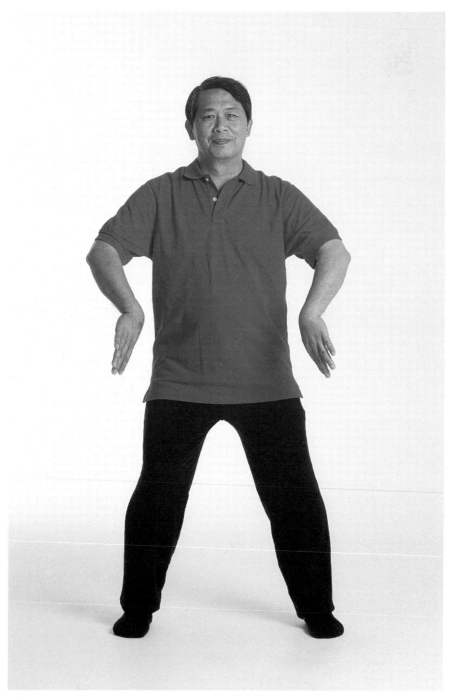

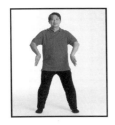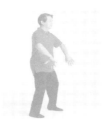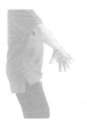

Holding

Standing Chi Kung practice is a natural progression from the seated practice. Since it is combined here with advanced positions of the arms and hands, you should only attempt this level of training after completing Level Two of seated Chi Kung practice shown in the chart on pages 46–51.

The placement of your feet is important since this is the foundation of the posture and your connection with the energy of the earth. Stand with your feet shoulder-width apart. You can check your position in a mirror. The mid-line of your foot is in line with the outer edge of your shoulder. Your feet point straight ahead. They are not angled outward or inward.

Begin this position with your arms by your sides. Then gently angle your elbows outward, away from your sides, letting your forearms be carried naturally along with the movement. Then rotate both forearms away from your body, so that your palms are turned outward to each side. Breathe naturally.

Follow the detailed advice about this position that follows on pages 122–5.

When you have finished your training in this position, gently fold your hands over your abdomen. Place your right hand against your belly and hold your left hand over it. Sit or stand still, holding your hands comfortably in place to lock your chi into your Tan Tien. Breathe naturally.

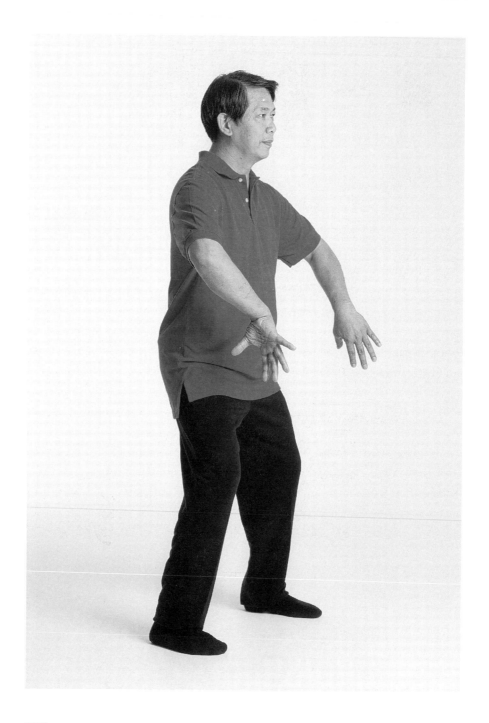

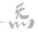

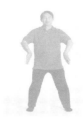 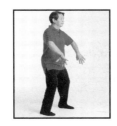 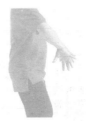

Holding

As you stand, relax your buttocks and hips. You may need to squeeze your buttock muscles and then release them to relax that area.

Lower yourself a little, as if you were about to sit down. This is a small, subtle movement. Do not sink too low – that will place too much strain on your hips and legs, especially if you are starting to practise Chi Kung for the first time.

Just feel that you are about to rest on a high stool. Feel your tailbone relaxing and descending.

You may slide down a couple of centimetres (an inch or so), but no more.

Your knees remain in place. There is no sense of kneeling forward.

You can imagine a large inflated ball being placed underneath your bottom to give you support.

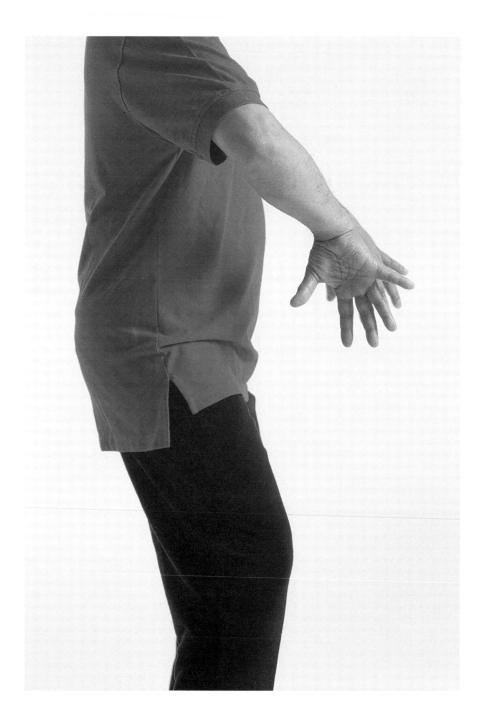

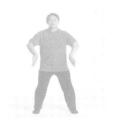 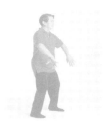 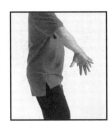

Holding

Your arms are to the sides, but are not pulled back beside your body. Your hands are just slightly in front of your body.

Your chest and shoulders are relaxed. Imagine large balloons supporting your arms in the space you have opened up under your armpits and upper arms.

Your palms are turned away to the sides, but are not twisted so far that they completely tighten the muscles in your forearms.

You feel that your elbows and forearms are naturally expanding outward, away from you. At the same time you sense that they are held within a large invisible sphere that completely surrounds you and holds you in place. This subtle sensation is the holding that occurs while you stand in this position.

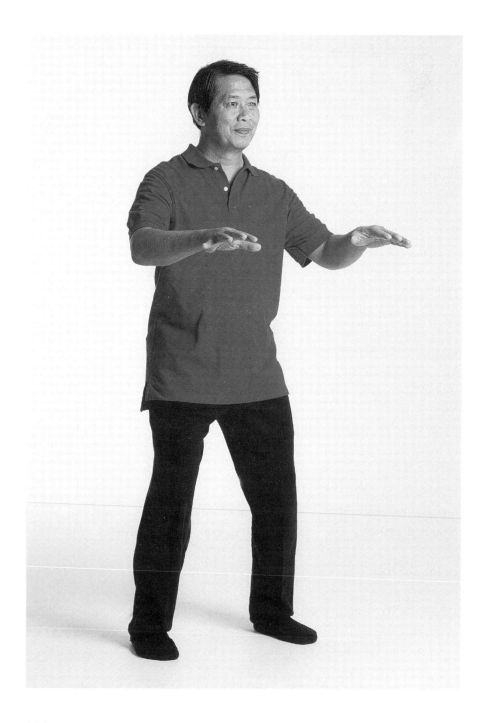

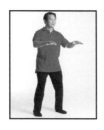 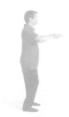 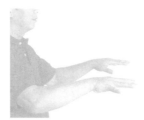

Expanding

As with all the positions in this section, you can practise standing or sitting. If you are standing, follow the instructions given for the second position, Holding, on pages 120–5. If you are sitting, be sure you begin by sinking your weight into the floor or seat. This position increases the energy developed in the initial stage presented on pages 52–57.

Imagine that you are holding the large balloon between your arms, with your hands level with the mid-point of your chest. The weight of your arms is supported by the balloons that you visualize under your armpits and forearms. Your shoulders and chest are relaxed. Remain in that position for a moment, to stabilize your energy.

Then turn your hands so that your thumbs point toward each other. Again visualize the balloons supporting your forearms and upper arms. You can also imagine that your wrists are held comfortably in place by a strap running around the back of your neck. Breathe naturally.

Follow the detailed advice about this position that follows on pages 128–31.

When you have finished your training in this position, gently fold your hands over your abdomen. Place your right hand against your belly and hold your left hand over it. Sit or stand still, holding your hands comfortably in place to lock your chi into your Tan Tien. Breathe naturally.

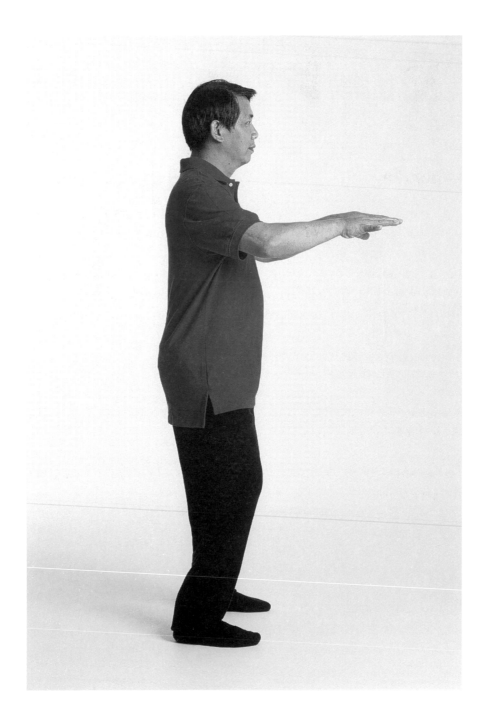

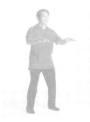
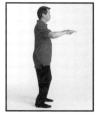
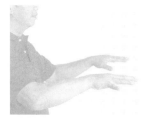

Expanding

The simplest way to move your arms and hands into the correct position is to begin with the original version of this practice shown on pages 52–7.

Begin by holding a ball in front of your belly. Then slowly raise the ball up in front of your chest, without hunching your shoulders. If your hands are at the correct level, the tips of your middle fingers will touch the mid-point of your chest if you fold them in to check.

Your wrists are slightly higher than your elbows.

Then simply rotate your forearms so that your palms turn away from your chest in the direction of the ground.

Your fingers are gently spread apart. Although they are relaxed, they are not drooping down.

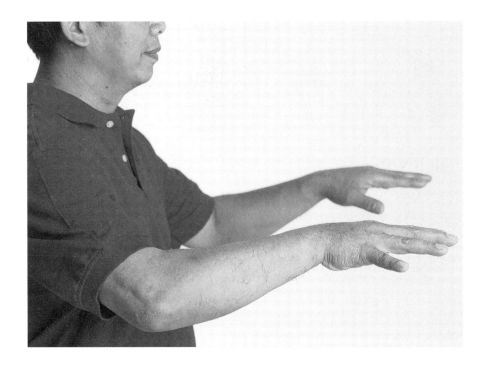

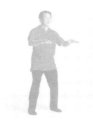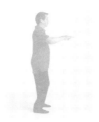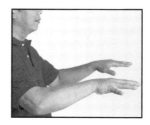

Expanding

As you stand with your hands in front of you, there may be a tendency for your shoulders and chest to become tense. You may feel a little aching or experience some trembling. This is natural since your body is more accustomed to relying on muscle strength to hold such positions, than allowing your internal energy to accomplish the task.

The secret is to make a deliberate effort to relax any muscles that seem to be tensing as you stand. So in the early stages of practising you may find yourself spending much of the time simply relaxing your chest and shoulders over and over again.

As you learn to relax, you begin to feel as if your hands are resting on top of a huge ball. It seems to be expanding upward and outward from within you. You may also begin to feel that your hands are expanding forward and that your neck is moving backward at the same time. As you relax into this practice, you will gradually experience these feelings and begin to understand the expansion that occurs. But if you try to force these feelings, you will be using muscle and creating strain that can hurt you.

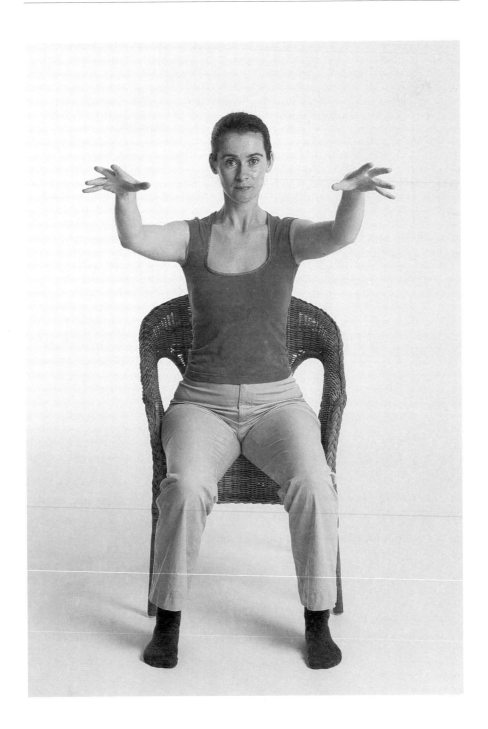

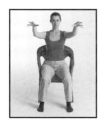 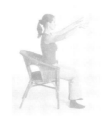 

Supporting

For most people this is the most demanding of the Chi Kung positions in this book. It is therefore important that you only attempt it if you have carefully followed the sequence of practices and instructions provided so far. You should have completed the structured daily programmes of practice outlined in the charts for Levels One to Five and completed all the previous stages of Level Six.

You can start practising this position while sitting if you wish, and then progress to standing. When you stand, your feet are shoulder-width apart. You lower yourself slightly, as if about to sit down. Then begin with one minute in the ordinary Lifting Position (pages 40–5).

Raise your arms into the original Supporting Position (pages 58–63), your hands turned away from your face. Stabilize in that posture for a minute. Pay careful attention, to make sure the muscles of your chest, shoulders and neck are as relaxed as possible. Then, keeping your arms in place, simply swivel your hands diagonally downward and outward so that your little fingers are as far apart from each other as possible. Breathe naturally.

Follow the detailed advice about this position on pages 134–7.

When you have finished your training in this position, gently fold your hands over your abdomen. Place your right hand against your belly and hold your left hand over it. Sit or stand still, holding your hands comfortably in place to lock your chi into your Tan Tien. Breathe naturally.

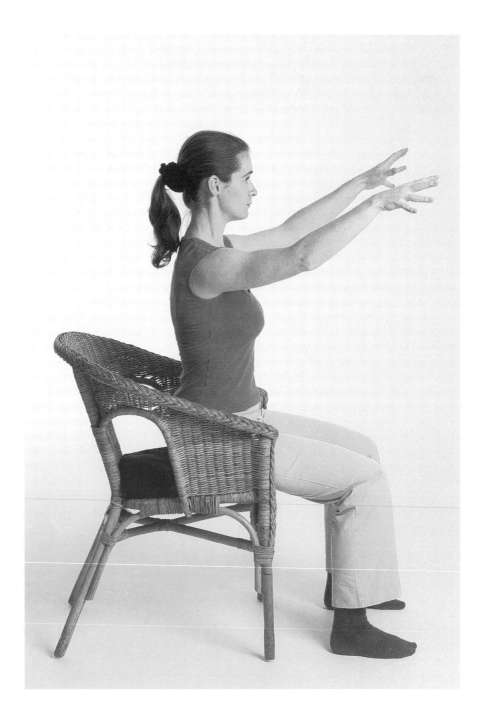

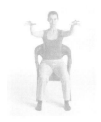 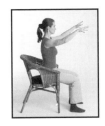 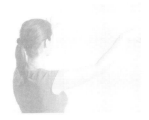

Supporting

In this position, your hands are further forward than in any of the other positions shown in this book.

Your arms extend almost directly forward, slightly opening diagonally outward.

There is a slight upward bend at each elbow.

Your wrists are higher than your elbows, level with your mouth.

As you hold the position, feel a constant sense of your shoulder and elbow joints opening and extending. Your upper arms extend forward, your forearms extend upward. These are invisible internal extensions. Externally, you are still and unmoving.

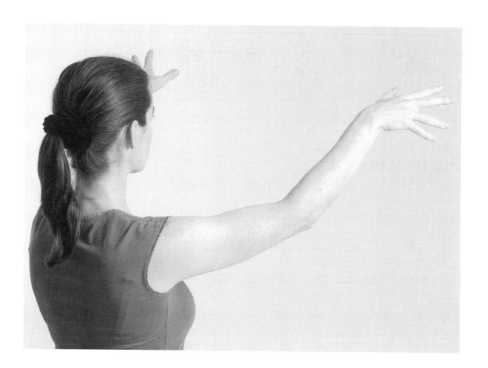

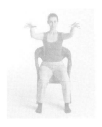
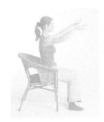
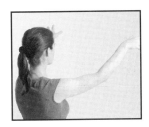

Supporting

This hand position is known in Chi Kung by the traditional Chinese term, Dragon's Mouth. Unlike the other hand positions shown in this book, the Dragon's Mouth involves deliberate and sustained stretching.

Moving your hands into position is like slicing outward through the air. Your little fingers and the blades of your hands lead the slice. Keep your hands at the limit of this slicing action, so that they are stretched horizontally outward.

Keeping your hands stretched outward, stretch your thumbs in the opposite direction, so that you feel the full spread between your thumb and little finger.

There is a further stretch within the Dragon's Mouth. Stretch the web of skin between your thumb and forefinger on each hand, by extending the forefinger.

There is a distinct feeling at the beginning of this practice that your energy is focusing outward from the 'mouth' on each hand formed by your thumb and forefinger, but as you hold the position, you experience a further sensation. You feel as if there is an invisible weight resting against your thumbs and forefingers. This invisible weight is supported by the architecture of your entire body from your feet, up through your spine and out through the back of your neck to your arms.

The deep power of this support comes from the earth on which you stand.

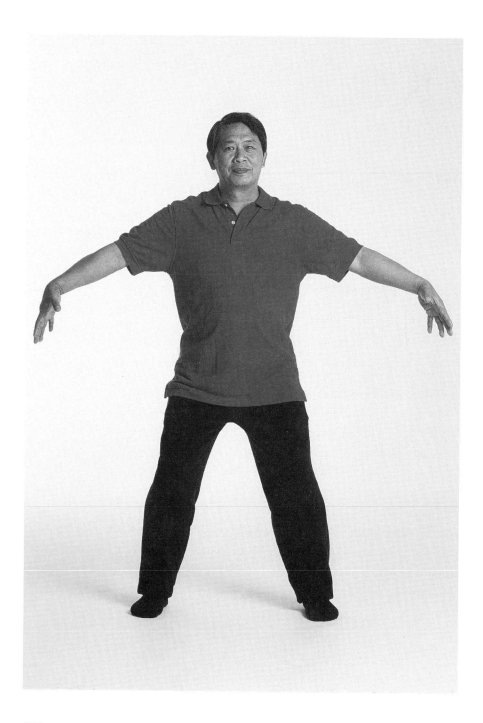

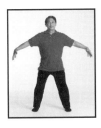 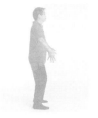 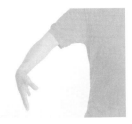

Floating

This is an advanced position that takes the original Floating Posture to a higher level of Chi Kung training.

You will experience the difference between the two levels if you start in the original posture with your arms extended to the sides, as if holding two balloons under each hand.

Then change the curve so that your elbows are slightly higher and your hands are lower than your wrists. You feel that the entire curved span of your arms rests on a huge balloon.

Breathe naturally.

Follow the detailed advice about this position that follows on pages 140–3.

Try holding this position in accordance with the graduated schedules given on pages 106–7. Once you have completed Level Six of your training, consult the sample schedules on pages 159–63 for advice on developing an advanced daily routine.

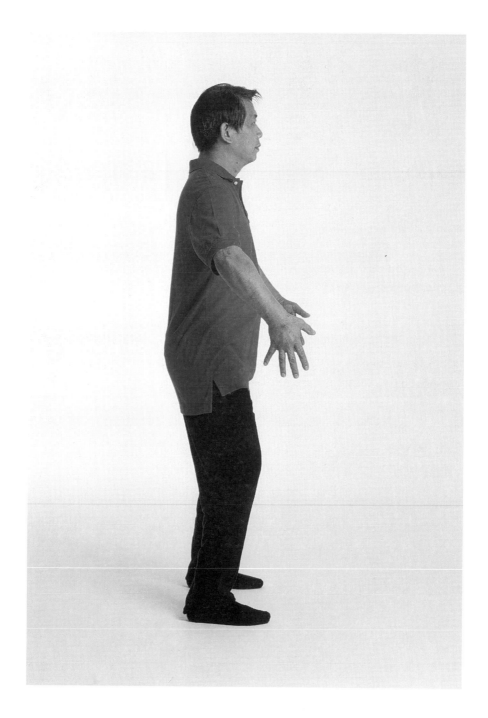

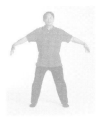
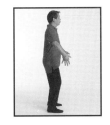
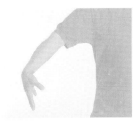

Floating

When you move into this position, be careful not to hunch your shoulders or pull them backward. Your chest and back should feel comfortable and relaxed.

As you can see from the photo on the facing page, your hands are slightly forward of the line of your body.

If you look carefully at the position of your arms you should be able to see two curves. First, there is the long downward curve from the shoulders to the fingers. Second, there is the gentle curve forward from the point where your arms connect with your torso out to your hands resting in space in front of your body.

Your fingers are gently spread apart and your palms are softly curved.

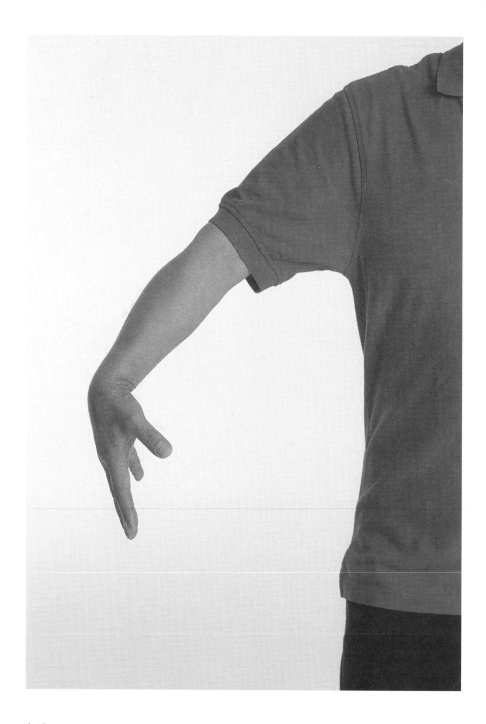

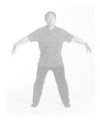 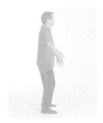 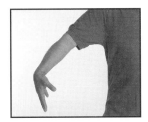

Floating

The simplest way to move your arms and hands into the correct position is to begin with the original version of this practice shown on pages 64–9.

You begin with your arms resting loosely by your sides and open your elbows outward. Then you lift your forearms up and out so that they are extended away from your body to each side. Your hands rest on imaginary balloons slightly forward of the line of your body. Rest in that position for a moment.

Moving into the advanced position involves adjusting the angles of your elbows and wrists.

First, slightly raise your elbows, keeping your shoulders in position.

Second, slightly angle your hands in toward your body.

Relax into this new position so that your shoulders, elbows and wrists are gently curved.

Your arm position has now changed into a long curve that feels like the reverse of the original floating position. Instead of holding two balloons while they float under your hands on a stream of water, you begin to feel that you yourself are one large balloon floating on a stream of energy, perfectly balanced and stable.

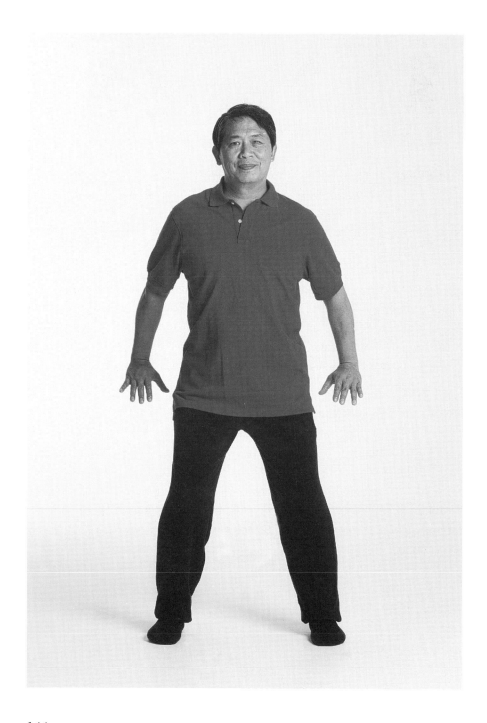

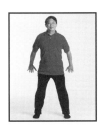
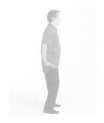
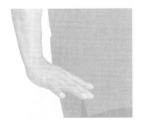

Pressing

Move slowly into the first position, Lifting, that you were introduced to on pages 40–5. Your elbows are away from your body and your hands are open beside your thighs. Stay still and relax into that position for a moment.

Then turn your hands so that the palms face downward and both hands are held parallel to the ground.

Draw your forearms slightly backward, so that the heels of your hands are in line with your hip bones.

Breathe naturally.

Follow the detailed advice about this position that follows on pages 146–9.

Try holding this position in accordance with the graduated schedules given on page 106–7. Once you have completed Level Six of your training, consult the sample schedules on pages 159–63 for advice on developing an advanced daily routine.

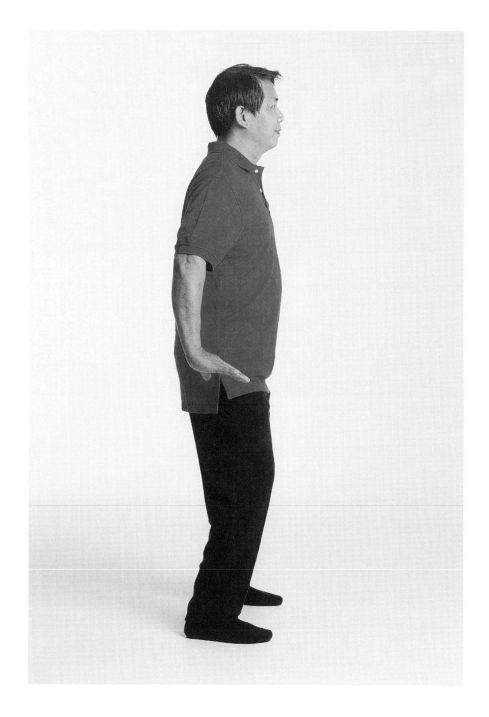

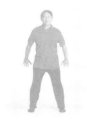 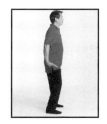 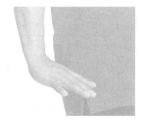

Pressing

When you draw your hands slightly backward, be careful not to strain your shoulders or chest. As you can see in the photo on the facing page, the hands are not pulled back beyond the midline of the body.

The elbows are angled outward from the body. They are not pulled straight back, as this would strain the chest and neck.

Feel the space that has opened up under your armpits. It is as if two balloons have been placed under your upper arms and are gently held in place by the natural circle formed between your upper body and your arms.

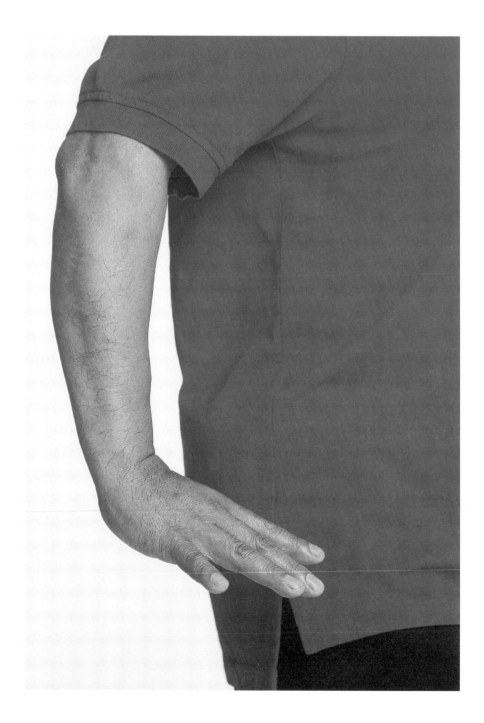

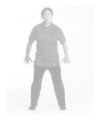 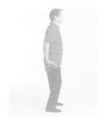 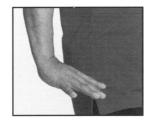

Pressing

Your hands are held parallel to the ground. The palms face downward. If you could extend your arms downward, your hands would be flat on the ground.

The fingers of both hands are gently spread apart.

Holding your hands in this way, feel a stretch in both wrists. It takes a little effort to keep your fingers open and extended. Try to keep both hands straight, as if you were gently pressing the entire palm and all the fingers flat on the floor.

As you gently press down with your hands, there is a natural response within your body. You feel your spine straightening a little and a sense of extension where your spinal column supports your skull. You feel the full power of your erect body expressing itself through the inner pressure of your palms. It is completely natural and must not be forced.

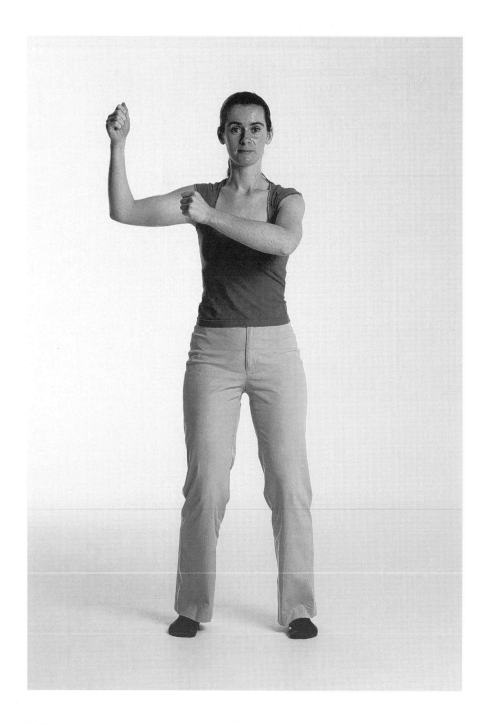

Hitting the drum

Now we come to the three concluding practices you should do after you practise these advanced Chi Kung positions. They help to release any tension that may have built up while you were training. They also unlock any excess chi that might have accumulated and store the extra chi you have generated in your Tan Tien.

To begin with, you need to dissipate any tension you may have built up in your upper body, shoulders and neck.

Stand with your feet shoulder-width apart.

Fold both your hands into loose wrists and bring them up beside your head on the right side. Breathe in as you raise your fists.

Then fling them down as if hitting a large drum in front of you. Breathe out sharply as your fists fly down on to the drum.

Then bring both your fists up beside the left side of your head, breathing in – and then fling them down to hit the drum again, breathing out.

Hit the drum twelve times.

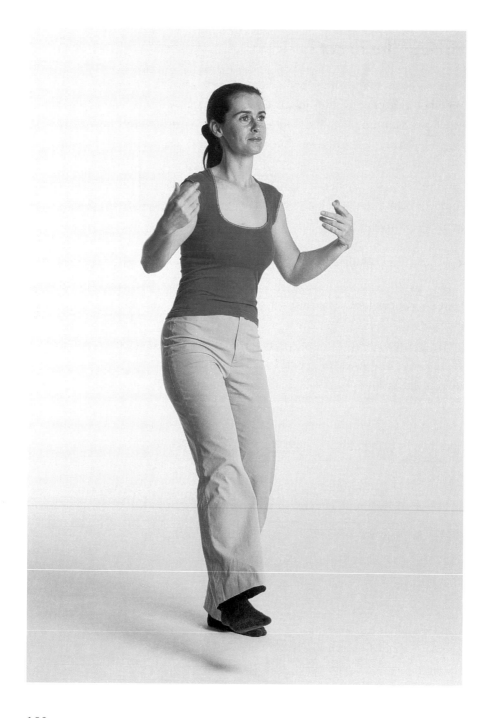

Shaking feet and hands

Whether you practise the advanced Chi Kung positions standing or sitting, you'll need to unlock any excess chi you may have built up in your legs or arms.

An easy way to do this is to shake your legs, one at a time, as if vigorously shaking sand off your feet. Make sure your whole leg is being shaken and that you feel the effects in your knees and ankles.

When you have shaken both your legs, then do the same to your arms. You can do them both at the same time, as if shaking water off your forearms, wrists and hands, with a series of continuous little flicks.

You can also try shaking both hands while shaking one foot and then the other.

Breathe naturally as you shake your feet and hands.

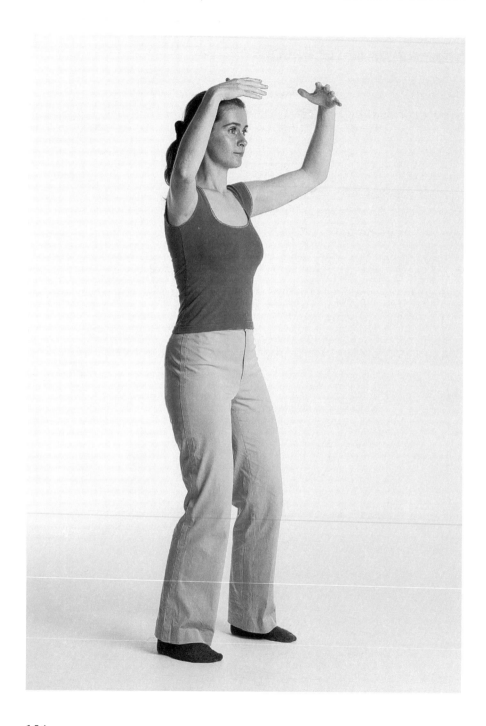

Circle down and sealing

This final movement directs your energy into your Tan Tien and seals it there. Always conclude your advanced training with this practice.

Raise both arms up beside your body in two large circles until your hands start to come toward each other above your head, but slightly away from the front line of your body.

Breathe in as your arms circle up.

Then slowly press your hands down in front of you, feeling you are pressing a large ball down into water. The movement continues until your palms have pressed down in front of your belly. Breathe out as your arms press down.

Then calmly fold your hands over your abdomen. Your right hand is against your belly, your left hand over it. Rest in stillness, breathing naturally for 30 seconds to a minute.

Chi Kung in Daily Life

As your Chi Kung practice develops, you will find many ways to add it into your daily life.

If you feel a little tired during the day, try doing any one of the 15-minute sessions suggested in this book. You may find that just doing the preliminary practices, which stretch your internal energy pathways and release tension, will make a noticeable difference.

If you are at work, or spend a lot of time sitting in front of a computer or at meetings, you can find lots of ways to do a little sitting Chi Kung practice. Often just sitting up straight with your hands subtly held in one of the positions for a few minutes will perk you up, mentally and physically. For example, if you are at a meeting, you can practise the original Holding Position, with your hands below the table in front of your abdomen (see pages 46–51).

If you are reading, hold the book or magazine, so that your elbows are away from your body and your hands are more or less in the Expanding Position, with the invisible ball between your arms and your chest. Your attention will be sharper and you will be much less likely to feel drowsy while reading.

If you are seated watching television, you can hold any one of the sitting Chi Kung positions for as long as you like. You can also take your training further by doing standing Chi Kung as you watch, although it is preferable not to do this during programmes that are violent or shocking.

If you are a sports enthusiast, you will find that Chi Kung practice is compatible with all other forms of exercise. It will give you increased stamina and greater resilience if you are injured. You will find the practices for Guiding your Chi (see pages 86–101) particularly helpful, as they strengthen the tendons.

In The Office

If you spend a lot of time in an office or sit a lot writing or working on a computer, try this sequence a few times a day. Sit naturally upright. Extend forward (pages 16–17) eight times. Follow this with the Expanding Position (pages 52–7) for a few minutes. Then do the corresponding movement for Expanding (pages 126–31). Follow this with Spread and Relax (pages 172–3) and conclude by resting your hands simply on the table in front of you.

Immobile

If you are bedbound or cannot move, try resting your hands over your abdomen, right hand on your belly, left hand on top. Tense and relax your calf muscles, first one leg, then the other, 36 times. This powerfully increases the circulation of chi and blood throughout your entire system. You can do this every hour if you wish.

If you fall ill or are recovering from an illness, you can do your daily Chi Kung practice while sitting up in bed, in a wheelchair or even while lying down. If you are able to sit up, then just follow the instructions in this book. If you are lying down, you will still find that you can do almost everything – if you lie on your back, it will be straight and you can follow the instructions as if you were vertical.

High blood pressure

If you suffer from high blood pressure, the Chi Kung positions that will help you are those that connect you with the energy of the earth and direct the flow of chi downward in your body. In the section, Building your Chi, these are the positions Lifting, Holding, Expanding, Floating and Pressing. In the section, Guiding your Chi, these are the movements, Holding, Expanding, Floating and

Pressing. In the section, Increasing your Chi, these are the positions Holding, Expanding, Floating and Pressing.

If you are hesitant about what to do, your practice can simply be the Preliminary Practices (pages 14–33), followed by the Lifting Position (pages 40–5) for up to eight minutes, followed by the Holding Movement (pages 46–51) 36 times, ending with the Concluding Practices (pages 114–19).

Low blood pressure

If you suffer from low blood pressure, the Chi Kung positions that will help you are those that connect you with the energy of the heavens and direct the flow of chi upward in your body. It is safe for you to practise all the Chi Kung positions in this book, as the combination of postures and movements will stimulate the flow of chi naturally throughout your body, including to your upper body and head.

If you are hesitant about what to do, your practice can simply be the Preliminary Practices (pages 14–33), followed by the Supporting Position (pages 58–63) for up to eight minutes, followed by the Supporting Movement (pages 127–37) 36 times. After this do the travelling exercise, Fearless Rider (pages 182–3), ending with the Concluding Practices (pages 114–19). Once you feel comfortable with this sequence, combine the Supporting Movement with the action of Fearless Rider so that you rise up and extend your arms and hands upward a total of nine times; then finish with the Concluding Practices (pages 114–19).

Creating your own practice

As you progress in your Chi Kung training you can explore the possibilities of 'mixing and matching' the different aspects of Chi Kung presented in this book: Building your Chi, Guiding your Chi and Increasing your Chi. Here is a sample 15-minute sequence drawn from those three stages of practice.

Seven-day patterns

Once you have completed your training from Levels One to Six, you can move on to other training schedules, such as this one, which covers a seven-day period. You may not always be able to train daily, but you can follow this sequence over a period of days if you wish, just picking up where you left off.

An alternative to this schedule is to train in the stationary postures from Day One to Day Six and then devote yourself on Day Seven to the movements of Guiding Your Chi (pages 86–101). You can either spend time on Day Seven training in just one of the six movements or you can build up to a higher level – training in all six movements in one session. As always, you begin and end with the Preliminary and Concluding Practices.

Day One	Always begin with the Preliminary Practices *(pages 14–33)* Lifting Position *(pages 40–5)* ten minutes Always end with the Concluding Practices *(pages 90–101)*
Day Two	Always begin with the Preliminary Practices *(pages 14–33)* Lifting Position *(pages 40–5)* one minute Holding Position *(pages 52–7)* nine minutes Always end with the Concluding Practices *(pages 90–101)*
Day Three	Always begin with the Preliminary Practices *(pages 14–33)* Lifting Position *(pages 40–5)* one minute Expanding Position *(pages 52–7)* nine minutes Always end with the Concluding Practices *(pages 90–101)*
Day Four	Always begin with the Preliminary Practices *(pages 14–33)* Lifting Position *(pages 40–5)* one minute Supporting Position *(pages 58–63)* nine minutes Always end with the Concluding Practices *(pages 90–101)*
Day Five	Always begin with the Preliminary Practices *(pages 14–33)* Lifting Position *(pages 40–5)* one minute Floating Position *(pages 64–9)* nine minutes Always end with the Concluding Practices *(pages 90–101)*.
Day Six	Always begin with the Preliminary Practices *(pages 14–33)* Pressing Position *(pages 68–73)* nine minutes Always end with the Concluding Practices *(pages 90–101)*
Day Seven	Always begin with the Preliminary Practices *(pages 14–33)* Hold each of the six positions for five minutes each Always end with the Concluding Practices *(pages 90–101)*

The Preliminary Practices Extending forward (pages 16–17) Side to side (pages 18–19) Double rubbing (pages 20–1) Gathering (pages 26–9) Sealing (pages 30–3)	**Essential to begin with these every day** • Extend your arms forward eight times • Turn from side to side eight times • Rub your knees 12 times • Hands in position 30 seconds to a minute • Hands in position 30 seconds to a minute
Building your Chi Lifting while seated (pages 40–5)	**Practice Times** Sit in this position for one minute
Guiding your Chi Holding movement while seated (pages 52–7)	**Practice Times** 36 times
Increasing your Chi Expanding while standing (pages 126–31)	**Practice Times** Stand in this position for nine minutes
The Concluding Practices Hitting the drum (pages 150–1) Shaking hands and feet (pages 152–3) Circling down and sealing (pages 154–5)	**Essential to end with these every day** 12 hits on the drum 30 seconds to a minute Hands in position 30 seconds to a minute

Reaching higher levels

Once you have completed Levels One to Six and have gone thoroughly through the seven-day patterns described on page 159–60, you can go further in your training. If possible, try to study with a qualified instructor. Otherwise, you can follow the suggested pattern below. At this stage, all your training will be done standing, holding the positions for longer periods of time.

The Preliminary Practices	Essential to begin with these every day
Strengthening the knees (pages 108–9)	• 12 rotations each direction
Rotating the hips (pages 110–11)	• 12 rotations each direction
Relaxing the shoulders (pages 112–13)	• 12 arm circles

The Six Positions – Standing	Practice Times
Lifting (pages 114–19)	Build up to standing in this position for 15 minutes
	Always include five minutes standing in this position when doing the remaining five positions as well
Holding (pages 120–5)	Build up to standing in the position for 15 minutes a session, one position in each session
Expanding (pages 126–31)	
Supporting (pages 127–37)	
Floating (pages 140–3)	
Pressing (pages 144–9)	

The Concluding Practices	Essential to end with these every day
Hitting the drum (pages 150–1)	12 hits on the drum
Shaking hands and feet (pages 152–3)	30 seconds to a minute
Circling down and sealing (pages 154–5)	Hands in position 30 seconds to a minute

If at any time you feel the level of energy is too much for you, slowly lower your arms, breathing out. Then do the Circling Down movement from the Concluding Practices six times, breathing out each time your arms pass down in front of you. Completely relax, sit down and rest.

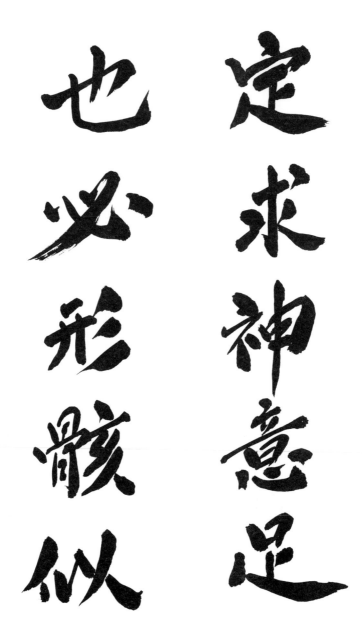

定求神意足
必形骸似也

CHAPTER SIX

RELAXING AND TRAVELLING

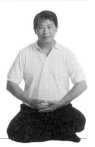

In this concluding section, you will learn more about one of the most important internal aspects of all Chi Kung practice – inner relaxation. It is often so difficult for us to relax in our busy lives, but learning to relax is the real secret of a healthy life. Even if you just take a minute or two to relax every couple of hours it can make all the difference. It's also useful to know how to relax after a busy day – the inability to relax is the cause of many sleepless nights.

This is where Chi Kung will make a real difference in your life. Chi Kung practice naturally relaxes you. That's what happens when you increase the flow of energy within your body. Even if you do just a little Chi Kung every day, you'll find you feel calmer. You'll start to notice that your nerves have become more steady. You will also start to find ways to use your Chi Kung training to create brief and powerful moments of relaxation at any time of your day.

Once you have got a feel for the inner relaxation practice, which is explained on the facing page, you will find that you can do it while holding all of the Chi Kung positions throughout this book. In addition, there are three exercises presented on pages 168–73, which you can use at any time to help you relax wherever you are and no matter what you are doing.

Travel tips

Most people I teach find themselves travelling at some point. For many, a long commute is a daily reality. Standing on railway platforms, at bus stops and in queues at airports provide golden moments for a little Chi Kung practice. Sitting on trains, buses, planes and boats also gives you time to undertake some practice. Most Chi Kung practitioners find little ways to practice without drawing attention to themselves. Feel free to experiment a little with the way you hold your hands in your lap, or possibly just slightly above your thighs, lightly inside your pockets or under a coat.

People often ask me what they can do on long flights to reduce the risk of thrombosis. Chi Kung is the answer! You can help yourself on flights or on other long journeys by doing the set of six exercises you'll find on pages

174–87. The alternating sets of tension and relaxation increase the flow of both blood and chi throughout your entire body. Try doing the whole sequence at least once an hour. You can go through the full set of exercises twice each time if you wish.

Learning to relax

Here is a simple relaxation routine to follow as you stand or sit in any of the Chi Kung positions. You can also follow this simple advice at any time of the day or night, no matter what you are doing.

Begin with the area around your eyes. Allow all the skin around your eyes to relax and imagine releasing any tension in your eyeballs.

Scan down to the angles of your jaw. Keep your mouth lightly closed, but make sure your tongue is relaxed. Be careful not to clench your teeth.

Let the feeling of release roll down the sides of your neck and over your shoulders, like oil. Let your shoulders slope downwards.

Breathe out gently, allowing your chest to relax.

Imagine a warm shower cascading down your back. Think of caked mud being softened and washed away by the clean water, starting with your upper back and moving down to your hips and buttocks. As an alternative, you can imagine cool air currents floating around you like a gentle breeze massaging your skin.

Feel the weight of your body descending onto your sitting bones or feet.

Then imagine a fine golden cord stretching from the uppermost point on your head up into the heavens. You feel your entire body is suspended from this point. As you experience this sense of suspension at the top of your head, balanced by the feeling of your weight descending as you sit or stand, scan your body for any remaining tension and gently release it.

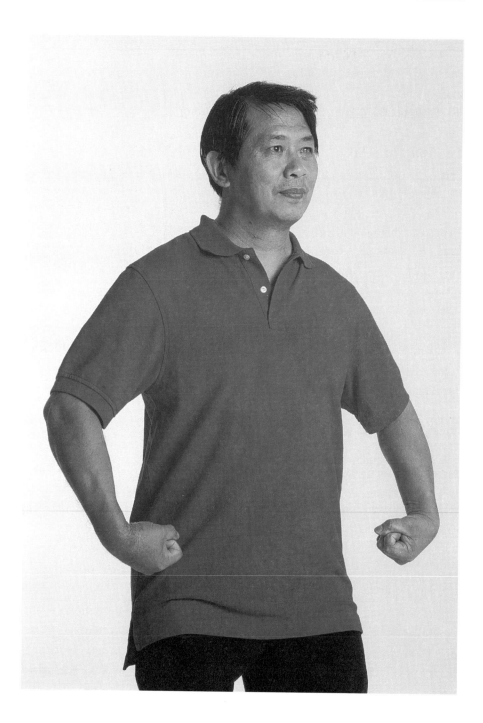

Clench and relax

Sit or stand upright if you can. This automatically releases pressure on your internal organs.

Let your arms hang loosely by your side for a second. Relax your shoulders.

Slowly open your elbows outward, away from your body, and move your arms into the original Lifting Position described on pages 40–5. The movement is led from the elbows, keeping the shoulders still. Your arms rest in an open, relaxed curve on either side of your body.

Breathe in.

Fold your hands into fists and clench them tightly while you hold your breath.

Hold tightly for a few seconds.

Open your hands as you breathe out, and lower your hands beside you.

Breathe naturally.

Repeat up to three times if you wish.

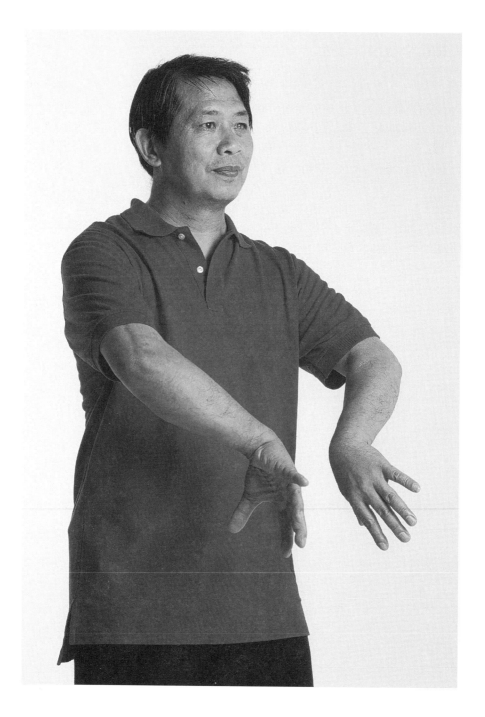

Twist and relax

Begin this relaxation practice with your arms by your sides. Then gently bring your hands toward your abdomen so that you are holding the large imaginary ball in front of your belly. Your elbows should be opened out, away from your torso, allowing space under your armpits.

Relax your chest and shoulders.

Breathe in.

Then rotate both forearms inward, so that the backs of your hands face each other. Breathe out as you do this. As your forearms turn inward, you may feel a slight twist in your upper arms.

Hold for a second. Breathe in.

Now clench both your hands and squeeze your fingers into fists as tightly as you can, and hold your breath as you do this.

Hold tight for a few seconds.

Breathe out, open your hands, return your arms to their normal position and rest your hands in your lap if you are sitting down.

Breathe naturally.

Repeat up to three times, if you wish.

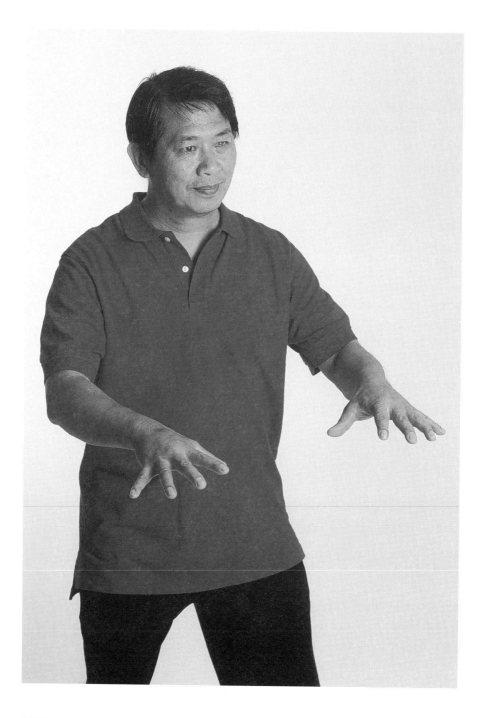

Spread and relax

Like all these relaxation techniques, you can do this standing or sitting. If you work at a computer or do other desk work, this exercise can be easily adapted to your needs: you can conclude by resting your hands on your desk, rather than your lap, if that is more convenient for you.

Begin by raising your arms, as if holding the large imaginary balloon between your arms. Imagine the weight of your arms being supported by the balloons that you visualize under your armpits and forearms.

Then turn your hands so that your thumbs point toward each other. Your palms face downward and your fingers point away from your body.

Breathe in.

Stretch your fingers and thumbs as wide apart as possible. The stretch should be as vigorous as possible, combined with a feeling that each finger is also extending forward.

Keep your fingers and thumbs spread apart for a few seconds, and hold your breath.

Relax the spread and breathe out.

Gently lower your hands to your lap or by your sides.

Breathe naturally.

Repeat up to three times, if you wish.

Travelling

Here is the full set of six inner exercises you can do when travelling. Each is explained in detail on the following pages, along with the inner visualization that arouses your chi.

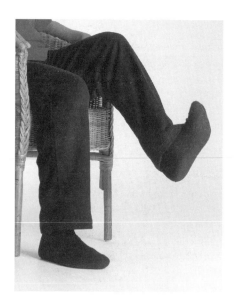

1. Giant Strides

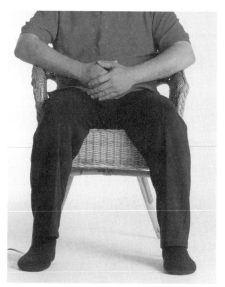

2. Bubbling Spring

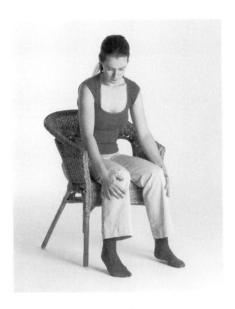

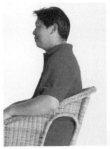

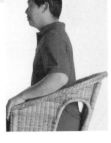

3. Waves on the Rocks

4. Fearless Rider

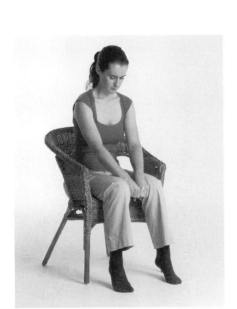

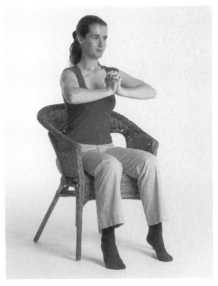

5. Crushing the Flanks

6. Holding Two Forces

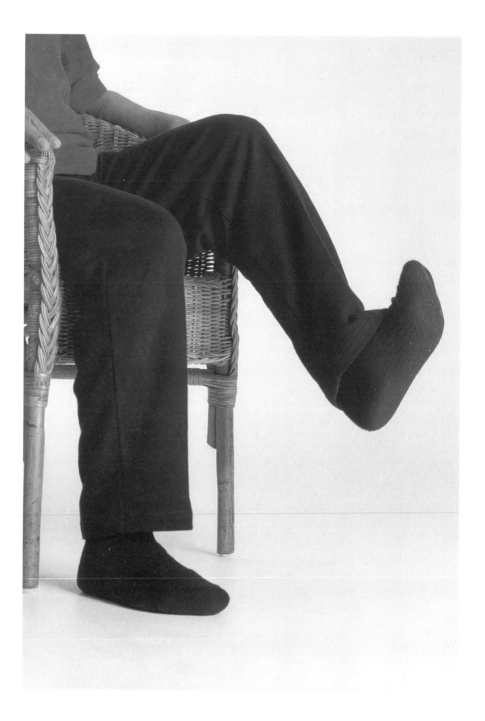

Giant Strides

Sit comfortably in your seat. If you can, straighten your back by sitting naturally upright. You can sometimes use the back of your seat or chair to help you straighten up without having to sit forward.

Slowly lift one foot off the ground. You can lift it 5 cm (2 in), or as far up as you can. As you raise your foot, also pull your toes up toward you as fully as possible. Breathe in as you raise your foot.

Slowly lower your foot as you breathe out.

Breathe in as you raise the other foot, also pulling your toes up toward you as fully as possible.

Lift your feet eight times. Wait ten seconds. Then repeat the sequence of raising and lowering two more times.

You can also do this exercise lifting your hands with each leg, as if your palms were pulling your legs up with invisible cords.

Imagine that you are taking huge strides over hills and mountains, like a giant. The movement is slow and powerful, your immense body covering miles with every step.

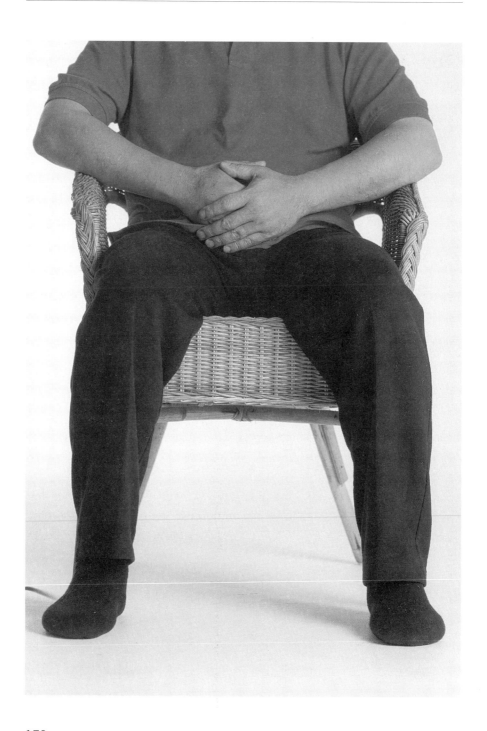

Bubbling Spring

This exercise is virtually invisible from the outside. Remain sitting comfortably in your seat. If possible try to keep your back as upright as possible.

Rest both your feet flat on the ground. Breathe in.

Then press the ball of one foot down into the ground. Try to use only your calf muscles to do this. Breathe out as you press the ball of your foot down for a couple of seconds.

As you press on the ball of your foot, you may allow your heel to rise up a fraction, but no more.

Relax, release the pressure on the ball of your foot and breathe in.

Then press on the ball of your other foot. Breathe out as you do this.

Press and relax eight times, first one foot then the other. Wait ten seconds. Then repeat the sequence of pressing and relaxing two more times.

As you press down, you are activating the Yung Chuan point on the sole of your foot, normally known as the Bubbling Spring. This action sharply increases the flow of chi throughout your system and the work done by your calf muscles speeds blood circulation.

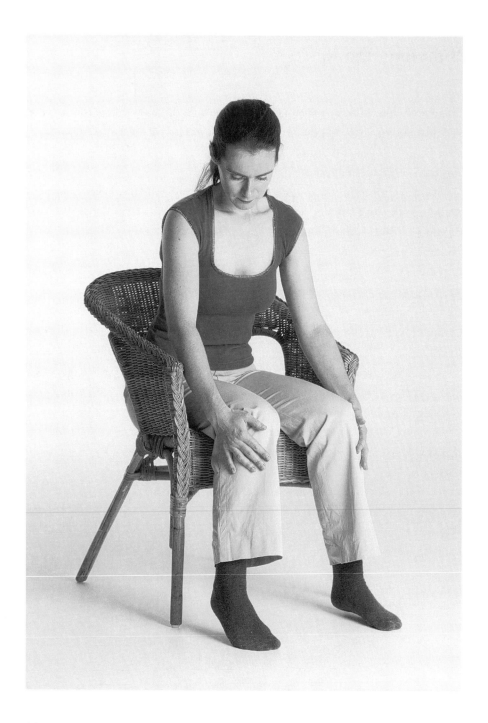

Waves on the Rocks

Place both your hands on your knees, so that your palms and fingers cover the entire area around the joints. Your fingers should curve over your knees so that your fingertips are well below your kneecaps.

Gently rub your hands in smooth circles around the whole of your kneecaps. Your hands should circle in an outward direction. The massage should be firm, but do not grip your knees.

Make 30 circles around the knees. If you have knee problems, do this massage as many times as you wish.

Breathe naturally.

To get the right feeling for this exercise, imagine that your knees are large rocks at the edge of the sea. Your hands flow around them just like waves rolling in, washing completely around them and then receding.

When you have finished, relax for a moment with your hands resting on your knees or thighs.

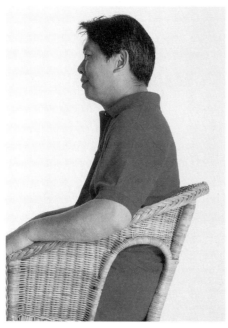

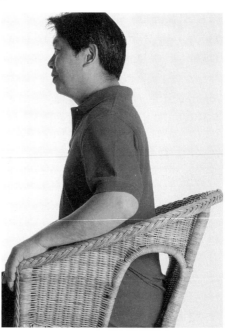

Fearless Rider

This exercise works best if you can sit forward in your seat or bring your back forward so that you feel yourself resting on your sitting bones. Your feet are flat on the floor.

Begin by resting back a little in your seat. Breathe in.

Then squeeze your buttock and thigh muscles so that they are as taut as possible and bring yourself forward so that you are sitting up straight. Breathe out as you come forward.

Hold the forward position for a few seconds. Your upper body is completely relaxed as are your calves and feet. The only work is being done by your buttock and thigh muscles.

Then gently release the pressure and completely relax as you breathe in. Rest back in your seat.

Sit up eight times. Wait ten seconds. Then repeat the sequence of sitting forward and back two more times.

You imagine that you are riding a powerful stallion. As you feel the horse about to leap, you pull yourself forward fearlessly to take the jump.

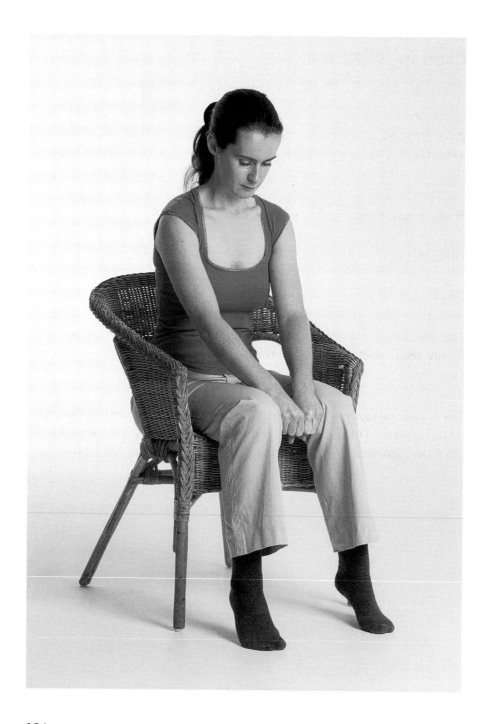

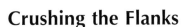

Crushing the Flanks

Sit forward if you can. Fold both your hands into loose fists and turn them palms downward. Bring your fists together so that the circle of your thumb and index finger on each hand touch each other. Place your fists together between your knees.

Squeeze your knees together, pressing inward on your fists.

Hold the squeeze for up to 30 seconds, if you can.

Breathe naturally.

You may prefer to do this exercise by pressing on your fists for ten seconds. Slowly relax. Wait ten seconds. Then repeat the pressing and relaxing two more times.

You are still riding the stallion. It is flying like the wind. To remain in position on its magnificent back, you need to grip its flanks between your knees. As you crush the flanks imagine the full power of the horse carrying you with it.

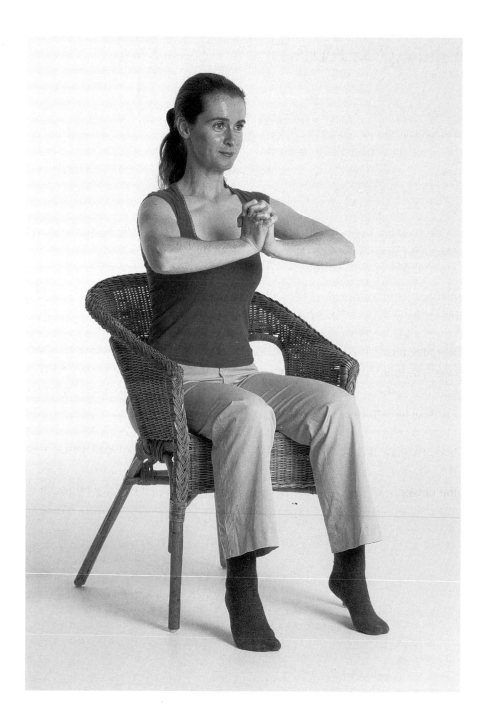

Holding Two Forces

Sit up as straight as you can in your seat. Slowly breathe out, letting your chest sink inward a little. Relax your shoulders.

Then, as you breathe in, bring your hands together in front of your chest and lock your fingers together.

Open your elbows outward so that your forearms form a right-angle with your hands. Your palms are now vertical, pressing against each other.

Now press your palms firmly toward each other as you breathe out. Keep pressing for 30 seconds while breathing naturally.

You may prefer to do this exercise by pressing your palms together for ten seconds while making one long exhalation. Slowly relax, keeping your arms in place. Breathe in slowly. Then repeat the pressing and relaxing with synchronized breathing two more times.

Your arms are like two forces relentlessly opposing each other. You feel the pressure they exert on each other, but your mind and body remain relaxed, so that the power of the two forces is calmly held by the entire field of your energy.

About the Author

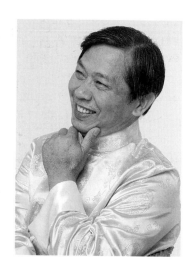

Master Lam Kam-Chuen is internationally renowned as a lineage holder of the art of Da Cheng Chuan Chi Kung, which traces it origins back some 27 centuries to the earliest foundations of classical Chinese culture. He has brought this art to the West and introduced the unique practices of Chinese health care to millions through his books and videos.

Master Lam began his formal instruction in classical Chinese arts at the age of eleven, training in Xing Yi under 80-year-old Master Fung, and subsequently learning the arts of the Northern Shaolin School under Master Lung Tse Cheung and Master Yim Sheung Mo. Both masters had been disciples of Grand Master Ku Yue Chang, at that time the 'King of Iron Palm' in China.

Also trained in Chinese medicine and having become a qualified herbalist and bone-setter, Master Lam opened his own health clinic and martial arts school in Hong Kong. As a member of the Hong Kong Chinese Martial Arts Association, he went on to victory in tournaments in Hong Kong and Taiwan and in the South-East Asia Open Tournament in Malaysia.

At this stage in his career he was introduced to a Yi Chuan master, trained in the tradition of Grand Master Wang Xiang Zhai, who founded the modern tradition of Da Cheng Chuan Chi Kung. This introduction led him to study in Beijing under Professor Yu Yong Nian, now the world's leading authority on this system.

In 1975, Master Lam, newly married to another martial artist, Lam Kai Sin, came to the United Kingdom. He accepted an invitation to teach Taoist Arts at the Mary Ward Centre in London, and has remained in the United Kingdom ever since. He continues to teach, and is nurturing the art of Chi Kung with a small number of The Lam Association's experienced students and teachers across Europe.

Master Lam is the author of a range of books on Chi Kung, Tai Chi Chuan, Feng Shui. Among his most widely read works, published in over a dozen languages, is his Chi Kung trilogy: *The Way of Energy, The Way of Healing* and *The Way of Power*. Television viewers will be familiar with Master Lam as the presenter of the ten-part Channel 4 series, *Stand Still – Be Fit,* now released as a Channel 4 video production.

For further study

If you wish to advance further in the study of Chi Kung, you should try to find a qualified instructor. This is not easy, and you will probably need to take the advice of a local Chinese medical clinic, if there is one in your area, or a properly accredited martial arts council. Even if you can't find a local instructor, you may find it helpful to continue your practice using three videos that give instruction and demonstrations of various aspects of the Chi Kung practices taught by Master Lam.

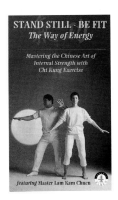

Stand Still – Be Fit

This is a series of ten-minute television programmes, each instructing you in the basic standing Chi Kung positions. They are filmed on location in China and presented by Master Lam.

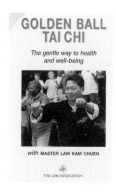

Golden Ball Tai Chi

This video takes you through two 15-minute sessions of exercise that includes Chi Kung and Tai Chi practices. It is specifically designed for senior citizens, filmed in London at a special open-air programme taught by Master Lam.

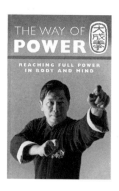

The Way of Power

This video is a unique presentation of the advanced practice of Da Cheng Chuan (The Great Accomplishment) for which the standing Chi Kung positions are the foundation. Filmed on location in China and London, it features both Master Lam and Professor Yu Yong Nian, the world's leading authority on this system.

To order these videos or to arrange an individual consultation with Master Lam, please contact him at:

The Lam Association
1 Hercules Road
London SE1 7DP
Tel/Fax: +44 (0)20 7261 9049
Mobile: +44 (0)7831 802598

For general information visit Master Lam's website at: www.lamassociation.org

Acknowledgements

Many people have made this book possible. First and foremost, I would like to pay homage to the masters with whom I have studied since my youth, and the long line of grandmasters and disciples stretching back over the centuries who developed and preserved the art of Chi Kung. I would also like to express my love and appreciation for my wife, Lam Kai Sin and to my three sons, Lam Tin Yun, Lam Tin Yu and Lam Tin Hun. They have all supported me in the long journey of transplanting this rare art to its new home in Western culture. This book was made possible through the efforts of one of my most devoted students, Richard Reoch, who has worked with me for many years to help share the wisdom of my own civilization with the rest of the world. Finally, I would like to thank Susanna Abbott, the commissioning editor at Thorsons, who invited me to write this book, was invaluable in the planning and editing, and kindly agreed to demonstrate many of the positions and exercises throughout the book.

Index